Rheumatoid Disease

Cured At Last!!

by
Anthony di Fabio

A publication of
The Roger Wyburn-Mason and
Jack M. Blount Foundation for
the Eradication of Rheumatoid Disease
AKA The Arthritis Trust of America®,
7111 Sweetgum Drive SW, Franklin, TN 37064
Original Copyright 1982

Preface

This book, *Rheumatoid Diseases Cured at Last!* was written in 1982 immediately after founding The Roger Wyburn-Mason & Jack M. Blount Foundation for the Eradication of Rheumatoid Disease, Inc.

Of course such a long title had to be shortened to either one of the two AKAs, The Arthritis Trust of America or The Rheumatoid Disease Foundation.

When money became available we funded serious medical research and thereby learned a great deal, but most of what we've learned since 1982 came through the activities of our then more than 200 referral physicians. Unfortunately most of our key medical partners as well as our brilliant Foundation medical advisor, Dr. Paul Pybus, has passed on. Subsequently most activities have been seen on our website at www.arthritistrust.org, where now thousands go to learn about how to get well.

In the past the ArthritisTrust of America's/The Rheumatoid Disease Foundation's cooperating referral physicians have successfully treated tens of thousands of patients afflicted with so-called incurable rheumatoid diseases using relatively low-cost, simple medical regimens.

The American Medical Association estimated some 13 million Americans sought relief from rheumatoid arthritis during one year. Three million were restricted in their daily activities. Seven hundred thousand could not do useful work, keep house, attend school or enjoy recreational activities.

Perhaps one out of every three people will suffer from some form of arthritis, and one person contracts the disease every 33 seconds. Dr. Carolyne K. Davis[1] of the U.S. Department of Health and Human Services stated that the U.S. Medicare program costs the U.S. Government about one billion dollars annually for rheumatoid diseases, and this was in the 1980s. Probably an equal annual amount is spent through State Medicaid programs, totaling U.S. Citizens about two billion dollars per year for treatment and care of those afflicted with the dreaded disease. At least one-half billion per year is lost in wages[2].

Others[3] estimated that 31 million Americans of all ages suffered from arthritis, that it attacks a million new patients a year, and did cost the national economy about

$1.5 billion annually[4].

For each male who suffers, there are three females. The symptoms often appear between ages of 20 and 35 with weakness, fever, loss of appetite and weight loss. One or more of the smaller joints becomes inflamed and swollen. Acute, painful inflammation migrates from one joint to another. Mental depression is common.

Attacks may develop gradually, or suddenly with dramatic seizure. Pain and inflammation may come and go for no apparent reason. The disease may affect children and produce stunting of growth and gross deformities.

Considering the insidious nature of rheumatoid disease, its many forms of symptoms and its long-term degenerative activity on your body -- sometimes extending from birth onward — apparently this book is for you, your relatives, and your friends!

1. Davis, K. Carolyn, Letter to Senator James Sasser, September 1, 1982, transmitted by letter to author by Senator James Sasser September 23, 1982.

2. *The Meridian Star*, "The Arthritis Foundation — Distributing Information to

Those with the Affliction," Meridian, MS, February 24, 1983.

3. *The Scanner*, Volume 1, Number 4, Fall 1981, The Arthritis Institute of the National Hospital for Orthopaedics and Rehabilitation, 2455 Army Navy Drive, Arlington,VA 22206, p. 1.

4. E. Harrison Clark reports that *Barron's* and *Wall Street Journal* report a figure of $1.5 billion, or a little less for pain-killers.

Chapter I
You and Your So-called Hopeless Disease
For the Rest of Your Life?

So, you've been told you have rheumatic arthritis, and there is no cure! For the rest of your life, you must watch your fingers and toes and arms and legs twist and turn and torture themselves into grotesque shapes that offend each eye and spirit!

When you awake each morning, your fingers and other joints are swollen, red and they burn as if held to a slow-roasting fire. You flex them and sharp pains make you grimace. Stiffened and puffy, your fingers feel like *not you*, like some burning, sausage-like appendages that were fastened on by instant glue during the night.

Gingerly protecting each joint, you slide carefully from your over-soft mattress. Oh, how it hurts to reach for clothing! Easy now! Not too fast, not too hard! Ouch! How that hurts! You wince, but go on dressing, though slowly. What else can you do?

The Ordinary Made Hard

Someone has tightened the coffee jar lid too much. A flash of resentment stirs as you wonder why others cannot understand, and why they cannot help you more by anticipating your weakness. Again pain forces your immediate attention. It's everywhere, at each joint — the terrible, long-lasting, daily increasing pain . . . .

Dare you risk injury to finger joints by fighting the coffee jar top this morning.

But you *need* the stimulation, the black, warm brew, something — anything — to lighten depression, to sway your outlook. . . .

So you struggle with the cap, gripping down on it, squeezing it and grimacing again, while sharp pains make you want to scream aloud -- and then-at last-the jar cap moves ever so slightly. Relaxing your fingers permits pain to diminish somewhat, and then you staunchly tackle the lid again.

You pour the steaming coffee ever so carefully and you hold it ever more gingerly. You must not place your fingers about the warm cup, for every finger joint will burn with a fury as though a small, hot laser beam were focused inside them. And so it is with cold items as well. Are you one of those who wisely insulates all cups and glasses?

Such are the once easy chores that now loom larger than life!

Perhaps you use special tools designed just for invalids with *incurable* arthritis: A wide-band holder for jar caps that multiplies weakened muscles and applies increased friction about the cap; a bathtub grip-bar (what a terrifying experience, that old-fashioned bathtub); an elevated toilet set; buttoning devices for shirts, coats, blouses; a special device for turning on and off kitchen or shower faucets (what an absurdly simple act that was once); long handles designed to reach clothing on the floor, and to permit ease in hanging them; special hooks and handles for special eye and needle affairs for tying shoe-laces — the mechanical devices are endless as the disease works into every musclefiber and joint.

Stiffness, Pain, Heat and Cold

How people comment about your hyperactivity! What they don't understand is that if you sit or stand or lay in one position overlong, you become stiff and your joints ache excruciatingly. So you move -- here, there, everywhere — all the time!

Do your hands and feet feel cold? Do you sweat night after night, with a terrible burning?

Your walking gait is changing; your skin bruises more easily and it has an increased fragility. Nodules have appeared in skin tissue, especially over points of pressure or friction. If you're bedridden the nodules will be found at the posterior portions of head, trunk and spine.

You might have developed skin ulcers or difficulties of another kind inside your lungs, or any of a dozen other physical problems that at first glance do not appear to be related to arthritis.

But you're probably one of the lucky ones, one of those who can still function, still determine your own physical course daily, still decide for yourself. What of those whose disease has progressed beyond, and now must lie bedridden, or rely on a wheelchair, and must be lifted and towed everywhere, must be dependent upon others, not daily, but hourly, for every little need, every little change, every little pleasure -- if any?

Are you still free and financially able to go to a warm climate where blessed relief may temporarily be yours? Oh, how cold rains and winds shrivel us and compress pain upon pain!

Hopelessness

Must you lie and stare, and hopelessly dream of the blessings of suicide, the relief of drugs, the wonderful numbness of alcohol . . . remembering that first visit to your doctor?

"You've rheumatoid arthritis and there is no cure. Oh, we know that within the first year you may have a spontaneous remission, that perhaps as much as ten to twenty percent of our patients get better. Although sometimes even those have it come and go again.

"Remember, it isn't true that nothing can be done for this disease. Aspirin will kill the pain, and when your system can no longer tolerate aspirin, we've indomethacin, phenylbutazone and many other drugs all designed very nicely to ease inflammation and your pain; we've antimalarial drugs like chloraquine and hydroxychloraquine, and sometimes we use gold compounds and/or penicillamine, although I wouldn't advise it personally; and there are several others, like propionic acid derivatives and tolmectin. . . .

"Then later, if you do not get better, we may give you cortisone shots — adrenocorticosteroids. I'd not advise that either unless very urgent, as there are dangerous side-effects . . . ."

Now that's how the old-fashioned doctors do it! What of the up-todate rheumatologists?

"I'd like to start you out with methotrexate. You know, the same cytotoxic drug that is used for treating cancer. It'll do no good, but then this substance is recommended."
[Gold compounds, penicillamine and cyto-toxic drugs

like methotrexate, aside from being useless, have never cured any rheumatoid disease and are believed to interfere with and diminish the effectiveness of The

8

Arthritis Trust of America/The Rheumatoid Disease Foundation treatment protocols by damaging the immunological system, and other bodily functions.]

"Don't fret because the majority of patients with rheumatoid arthritis can continue to lead active lives with varying degrees of restrictions. We must not seek a short-term solution, but plan for long range management of your problem.

"There are no specific dietary recommendations[1], but you should maintain a good balanced diet with the four food groups, and there are no indications of vitamin supplementation, unless, of course, you just happen to have a special vitamin problem, which I don't believe is true for you." [This statement is false. Proper nutritional support and vitamin-mineral supplementation is known to be vital to altering the course of arthritic problems and returning the patient to health.]

"Weight reduction — and keeping it off — should have a high priority.

"You must have rest, and we must determine a program of maintenance of joint function by standardized physical measures, and also we don't want your muscles to atrophy. In other words, some kind of exercises are a must, so long as you don't over-stress your joints.

"Then there is the inevitable depression and fatigue. . . ." "Depression?" you ask. "Fatigue?"

Do you need a lecture on depression and fatigue? Sharp and dull pains bombard your each waking

moment, until there is nothing left but for your analytical mind to attenuate, to close down, to push you into a state of emotional apathy that is beyond words.

Nothing, absolutely nothing on earth or beyond earth, can have meaning when you are at lowest ebb. Loved ones speak, and you groan, or turn-over, or at the very best you growl out, "I just don't give a damn!" and you mean it with every cell, every fiber of your being. Your spouse could move out at that instance, and you'd care not! Your beautiful children could be crying of ache and loneliness, and you'd care not! You could be told of inheriting a million dollars, and you'd care not! A flying saucer could land beside your bedroom window emitting five little green men, each carrying strange weapons that will evaporate anything they touch, and you'd care not!

You could die at that instant, and you'd care not! Please physician, tell us about apathy and fatigue. . . .

Traditional Treatments

But the body recovers with rest, although with lessened vigor at each interval, and morning comes again. You struggle to dress, to remove the coffee jar lid, to move about, and to bathe and go through the motions of easing your daily load.

Time passes. Another trip to the doctor -- and another. Your medicine closet bulges: besides aspirin there is now Indocin®, Butazolidin®, Motrin®, Clinoril®, Tolectin®, Naprosyn®, Feldene®. Each day you

take one or another with increased frequency.

You may be one of those whose system rebels further, and you may suffer eternal diarrhea, or you may have developed stomach ulcers, or some other insidious problem — just when you thought your body withstood all the problems it could bear . . . !

Little by little, over weeks and months, you watch fingers and toes turn and bend, despite rigorous exercises, and you constantly fight pain. There is absolutely nothing that can be done, except now and then expensive physical therapy might slow the terrible deformation if conducted under proper professional conditions — but eventually nothing helps when the very joints and cartilage and tendons themselves have been eaten alive.

Now you've become a ranking candidate for prosthesis, those wonderful steel and plastic devices that are transplanted into joints.

Terrible you say?

Not so! Not if your life consists of unmoving, continuous staring at a colorless, lifeless ceiling above your bed, and a terrible moment by moment waiting for someone to come and move you from hither to thither.

Joint by joint is destroyed by the raging inferno of your own immunological system, your life eating up yourself, and joint by joint can, perhaps, be replaced, until there is little of you left at all, or until you finally, blessedly, succumb to the greatest depression of all — death!

You are probably intelligent enough to know your future — you've seen so many others with this terrifying sickness. You've got choices. You can fight, do all the things your family doctor tells you to do: keep down inflammation and pain; exercise, but also rest frequently.

Non-traditional Treatments

Or, like so many of us, you can ignore futile medical science and irrelevant technical knowledge and react to hearsay, superstition, panaceas. You know! Copper bracelets[2]; cactus juice[3]; special diets; faith healers; mumbo-jumbo of one kind or another.

Who can blame us?

There is no hope, because traditional medical doctors have told us there is no known cure. And every day the depression and pain and fatigue and weakness increases, as does the bending and twisting and distortion of ourselves.

You look in the faces of loved ones, spouses and children and grandchildren, who move with gay abandon and carry on life with zest that was once yours — and you wonder — can you impose this frightful crippling burden on their wonderful future? Do you have the right? Do they have the obligation to suffer with you?

What kind of terrible sin have you committed, you secretly wonder, that the Lord put this on. . . .

Somewhere secretly deep inside you've committed yourself to ending it all at just the right time if you can find a way to do so without hurting them.

Meanwhile, seize any hope -- something is better than nothing at all, even if that something is simply fantasized hope! Who would take that away also?

So there is nothing you can do!

Live with it, and search for relief anywhere, everywhere, and hope or give up life completely — that's your choice!

So we search in national newspapers for special arthritis cures — if you don't like this week's, there's always another coming along next week just to keep our fantasies alive; we look into fancy diet books and magazines and organic health journals; we carefully listen to positive sounding, authoritarian faith healers, those men who are so sure that if we will just "believe" then a higher power will reach out with a mystical touch and lo! we are healed; oh, how we donate to their favorite causes; and we drink this briny juice, or eat that tasteless herb, or we go on special diets that would normally make us very happy if we were herbivores; or we spend time and much money getting ourselves analyzed and explained away by one school of head-shrinks or another. . . .

No matter, all the time the terrible fires rage, our joints puff and shriek with pain, and the inexorable horrible twisting and turning joints distort onward!

So Where From Here?

So here you are now, with this publication, with just another claim to cure. You're pessimistic, aren't you? You have a right to be. So, keep your pessimism.

If what follows makes sense, you'll try it, like you've tried so many other things that didn't work, even when they didn't make sense. If it is science, if it is proper medical practice, it'll work. If it works, you'll be well. If it doesn't work, you're no worse off, especially since the time and cost involved in this alleged "real cure" is relatively tiny, and especially since your own family doctor can be party to the cure.

What have you to lose? A six weeks -- perhaps several additional months -- trial at very little cost under your own family physician?

That's not much compared to an endless lifetime draining cacti of their sap, or eating alfalfa, or doing some other silly thing, is it? [Distrust of these traditional folk remedies have turned into appreciation of many of these approaches for good reasons.]

Read on, if you dare, if you can stand one more hope. And God be good to you as he has already been good

to so many others. . . .

1. Advice from some physicians differ. Dr. Robert Bingham, for example, states that 60% of rheumatoid arthritis patients have dietary deficiencies, and 80% have

vitamin and mineral deficiencies.Most doctors associated with The Arthritis Trust of America/The Rheumatoid Disease Foundation would increase both categories to 100%.]

2. According to Professor Roger Wyburn-Mason, copper ions from a copper bracelet, on invading the bloodstream, can in fact weaken an amoebic infection which he felt was the primary source-cause of rheumatoid arthritis; but that the copper ion concentration from a bracelet source is not usually sufficient to reduce the infective population in the drastic numbers necessary. Later, Professor Wyburn-Mason seemed to demonstrate that pure metallic copper ions in stronger concentrations did constitute an effective treatment for many people. See "The Use of Ionic Copper in the Treatment of Arthritis," Seldon Nelson, D.O., The Arthritis Trust of America; republlished from *The Journal of the Academy of Rheumatoid Diseases,* Vol 1, No 3,

3. According to Dr. Robert Bingham, Yucca juice is helpful for some rheumatoid arthritis patients. Its usefulness seems to come from its two most important chemical components: saponin, which facilitates the combination of oil and water aiding digestion and elimination, the other, a vegetable steroid related to the cortisone family of drugs, thereby relieving symptoms.

Yucca has also been shown to have broad-spectrum antimicrobial effects in water treatment and has reversed arthritis in horses, according to Stephan Cooter, Ph.D.]

Dr. Jack M. Blount's (M.D.) "Miracle"
Dr. Jack M. Blount's Gift to Mankind
Dr. Jack M Blount's story is an emotionally gripping account of a man who has been to the very depths of hell

and has come back to tell us how he escaped the fires. He tells his story simply, without any attempt to embellish, and it is told with a genuineness that makes you believe in his continued concern for your health and welfare.

In this chapter Dr. Blount will tell his own story in his own words. Keep in mind that he is cured of the ravages of rheumatoid arthritis, that he has since treated better than

16,000 patients successfully, and that he freely gave of his knowledge to any who asked.

He is a man who was active physically in his youth although his symptoms began as a systemic illness in his teens with muscle pain, pain in the foot (metatarsalgia), lumbago (pain in the back), intercostal (between ribs) pains, inflammation of eye (iridocyclitis), psoriasis (skin lesions) and that eventually he got pains in the joints, generalized arthritis with effusions (fluids into joints), carpal tunnel syndrome (compression of nerve in wrist), paresthesia (loss of feeling or perverted sensation), ulcerative colitis (sore or inflammation of colon), aseptic necrosis (death) of a femoral head for which a prothesis (steel and plastic joint) was inserted, etc. He was reduced to total invalidism and took to alcohol, morphine-containing drugs, barbiturates and was a terminal case. He had to give up his medical practice in March 1974 after having taken steroids for the pain of Rheumatoid Arthritis for more than twenty years.

Dr. Blount's Story: Rheumatoid Disease is of the Entire Body

I cured myself and more than 16,000 others of an incurable illness. "Rheumatoid Arthritis." I call it a MIRACLE.

I had rheumatoid disease. Rheumatoid Arthritis is a disease of the entire body, not of just the joints although most of the pain and destruction seems to be in and around the joints. I was hopelessly ill.

In the Spring of 1974 I had developed aseptic necrosis (complete destruction) of my right hip socket and femoral head. I had to quit work (private medical practice) and take to bed. The only thing that would help was a hip replacement with a prosthesis. The orthopedic surgeon that I went to said at first he would do the operation but then changed his mind giving the excuse that because I was only fifty-two years old at the time I was ineligible. They didn't know, yet, how much dependence to put on the procedure.

Despair

Despair set in, I could only lie in bed and stare at the ceiling. The cure of my illness was hopeless. No one knew the cause. No one know anything useful to do for it. The usual advice was to take a lot of aspirin and learn to live with it. Pharmaceutical companies tried to improve on aspirin and gave us Butazolidin®, Indocin®, Motrin®, Tolectin ®, Nalfon® , Naprosyn ®, Clinoril® , Meclomen®, etc. They called these "nonsteroidal anti-inflammatory" agents [NSAIDS]: all were useless except for some analgesic effect.

"Cortisone" was introduced in 1949 and was hailed for a while as the long awaited answer. It was, and still is, the quickest relief of arthritis symptoms, but it causes devastation worse than the disease. These adverse effects included hyperadrenalism (Cushing's Disease) diabetes, ulcers, weakened bone, (decalcification) etc. I took a form of this for about twenty years.

While lying in bed my arthritis became complicated by colitis, with diarrhea of sometimes up to twenty times a day, kidney stones, alcohol, and drugs. I was in and out of hospitals repeatedly. I thought I would surely die. Friends kept sending word that they were praying for me. I often thought of committing suicide. The pain and agony was unbearable. One morning after I had accumulated about forty Seconal® capsules (sleeping pills) I swallowed them all. Four have been known to kill. I didn't want to kill myself, but I couldn't endure such perpetual agony. After some hours my wife found me unconscious and on finding the empty bottle, she knew what I had done. I awoke very groggy and tied to a hospital bed. After regaining enough sense to know anything at all, I wanted to know if I had been apneic. (Had I been deprived of oxygen long enough to cause permanent brain damage?) I was assured the answer was "no." Despite such an overwhelming dose of sleeping pills I had continued to breathe adequately without supplemental oxygen or assisted breathing. This was a miracle in itself. "Somebody up There" was not ready for me.

Why Was I Saved?

Back home I kept breathing but hardly living. Why was I still here at all? I had been waiting for some earthly savior and none came. Was there some "learned University professor or researcher" somewhere who knew something to do?

The Miracle of

Professor Roger Wyburn-Mason

One day in the spring of 1976 I came across an article in *Modern Medicine*[1] entitled "Rheumatoid Disease: Has One Man Found the Cause and Cure of Rheumatoid Disease?" written by Robert Bingham, M.D., practicing in California. Dr. Bingham, orthopedic surgeon, had heard of work done by Professor Roger Wyburn-Mason, M.D., Ph.D., England, and had gone there to interview the

Professor. His article told about how the English researcher, practitioner, microbiologist, had determined that the etiological agent (cause) of rheumatoid disease is actually a germ, a protozoan, an ameoba, similar to the "lettuce bug" amoeba that causes dysentery. He also reported that a chemical (in fact, several chemicals) had been found that would kill the "bug" in patients without killing the patient.

He was curing people who had the disease that was killing me. The chemical (medicine) that the Professor was using successfully was called clotrimazole[3].

That's wonderful, but how could I get some for myself? It was not on the market anywhere in the world for systemic use.

Finally, in the Spring of 1976, my orthopedic surgeon decided to operate. They removed the upper part of the right femur with the femoral head and reamed out the acetabulum (socket). The socket was filled in with plastic to make a new one and the bone was replaced with a "comma-shaped" steel rod with the pointed end inserted down into the marrow, distally (farthest from center or medial line), of the remaining femur.

Now, I thought I would recover. But recovery was terrible. I still needed my pain medicine and booze. My brother became disgusted with me and had me sent to an alcoholic ward and "detox" center at the State Hospital. After a month there I was off everything addicting except my daily early morning "Cortisone." I still had my rheumatoid disease -my germs, the amoeba. I still had to rid my body of them. The operation seemed to give them new life.

Somehow, I remembered that clotrimazole is the active ingredient in a preparation used to treat yeast and fungus infections of the skin but it was just one part clotrimazole plus ninety-nine parts propelene glycol, car antifreeze — Prestone®. This is poisonous to man if taken internally.

I decided to telephone Delbay, the company that puts the mixture together, and see if I could get clotrimazole that hadn't been mixed. The answer was "no." They were afraid of the U.S. Food and Drug Administration.

Failing with that endeavor I started wondering if there might be something else almost the same that would work. I looked at the word 'clotrimazole' and focused on the 'azole'. I looked that up in the medical dictionary and found that the parent of this is 'Imidazole'. Somehow I remembered that I had heard that word somewhere before. I kept repeating it. Then I remembered that this is the chemical name of the medicine metronidazole, or Flagyl®. I compared the formulas of the two and they looked close enough alike that I thought it was worth a trial. We [Americans] had had Flagyl® since 1962 and used it to cure amebiases (intestinal) and vaginal trichomonas infections [as well as vaginal yeast infections]. It was known to be able to kill both of these protozoa. I decided to try it. Later I pulled out a drawer in my bath room and there was a bottle of one hundred Flagyl® tablets. A MIRACLE! God had put the answer to my illness that close to me.

How should I take it? I realized that the small dosages that were recommended for trichomonas and intestinal amebiasis [and yeast] would not do any good. If it would have, someone would have discovered it accidentally. I checked the medical text books and saw that it had been given in doses as high as three tablets, 250 mg, three times daily. That is the amount I started to take.

I Experiment On Myself

I didn't know how long to continue taking it. I didn't know if it would kill me. I realized I didn't have much to lose; therefore I took all I had which lasted eleven days. On the morning of the eleventh day, I got nauseated while brushing my teeth -- nd emptied my stomach. Then I knew I couldn't take anymore even if I had had more readily available, so I stopped. [This early experimental dosage is not recommended. See The Arthritis Trust of America/ The Rheumatoid Disease Foundation protocol for correct dosages by body weight[17].]

But during these eleven days a miracle had begun to happen. My arthritis started getting better. I awoke in the middle of the night and realized that the soreness, stiffness, and swelling had started subsiding. I looked at my hands which had been so bad and now were so much better. I couldn't hold back the tears. I started praying and thanking God.

After that I didn't know how much was enough. I knew that I was still sick. I still had sweats and felt cold. I was bound to still have the infection. After two weeks I decided that I needed more. I restarted taking three 250 mg tablets three times a day. I took it for eleven days more and on the eleventh day I got nauseated again. But, I was surely improving by the day. I decided to continue this pattern.

More Successful Patients

I decided to find out if some of my former arthritis patients were brave enough to try it.

I telephoned them and invited several of them to my home, one at a time. To each I explained what it was all about. Every single one was eager to try it, nothing else had ever helped. Why not? During the Summer of 1977 about thirty of them were treated and most of them had the same good experience that I had. Some got nauseated from the start and decided to quit.

Among the thirty was a Reverend Ethel Beall. Brother Beall not only had arthritis, but had lost a leg due to an automobile accident. The bone in the stump of the leg had gotten infected and drained constantly and was always painful. During this treatment period with Flagyl® his arthritis got better and his leg got well and stopped hurting. (Several months later he died suddenly of embolus [blood clot] while recovering from a prostate operation).

Well Again!

After 8 months I was able to return to my private medical practice on a limited basis. I had been out three and one-half years. On September 1st 1977, I was back in the office seeing patients by appointments.

I decided to write Professor Roger Wyburn-Mason in England and tell him of my experiences. I owed him my life. He answered immediately and said that he had decided to include my case in a book he was writing. *The Causation of Rheumatoid Disease and Many Human Cancers — A new Concept in Medicine.* My story appears on page 205 in the book[2].

We continued to correspond and I visited with him during the Summer of 1978. He told me that he tried metronidazole at one time and it didn't work. His dosage was not adequate; he had tried giving only 250 mg three times daily. However, later he gave 750 mgm three times daily and it did work about equally as well as clotrimazole. He found other nitroimidazoles that would do the job, also. [This dosage is not recommended. See The Arthritis Trust of America/The Rheumatoid Disease Foundation protocol for correct dosages by body weight[17].]

Later he found three commonly used medications that are ameobicidal when used in high doses: furazolidone, allopurinol and rifampicin. [There are also others[17].]

His experiments proved that Flagyl® and the other nitroimidazoles are excreted slowly from the body and it is not necessary to give them on a daily basis. After giving a loading dose for two days there is an effective blood level (for killing the amoebae) for several days more. During the past six years I have treated more than 16,000 arthritic people with very gratifying results. Some are cured of the disease while in others it has been arrested. (People were coming from all over to share in the miracle.) Professor Roger Wyburn-Mason should have beeen nominated for the Nobel Prize in medicine.

Prayer for the Entire World

I pray that the entire world will soon know and people every where can receive the same relief that I have. What a joy I know now!

I thank God!

This information is free to whomever will take and use it. I need no wealth and seek no fame.

Important Note

William Renforth, M.D. (Connersville, IN, USA) deserves respectful praise for research of nitroimidazoles prior to 1977, distributing information and pioneering in the use of metronidazole for treatment of Rheumatoid Disease.

Dr. Archimedes Concon, (Memphis, TN), following a non-amoebic theory, also effectively used metronidazole for Rheumatoid Diseases prior to 1976[4] .

Professor Roger Wyburn-Mason died June 16, 1983. As of 1996, Jack M. Blount, M.D. was still free from

Rheumatoid Arthritis and conducted a limited private medical practice. He died later of liver problems.

Anthony di Fabio is Also Cured

The Beginning of Arthritis

In 1978, at age 53, I began suffering from the first pangs of rheumatoid arthritis, although at the time I passed it off as simply unimportant, transitory pains in toes, fingers and groin of unknown origin.

By choice I slept on a hard, cotton-pad, but slowly my shoulder pains became so great that foam padding had to be overlayed.

Later visits to medical specialists brought out that the pains were from "degenerative arthritis." This diagnosis was "confirmed" by medical doctors at the Veteran's Administration Hospital.

Fatigue and Depression

During the following year I began experiencing a kind of fatigue that sapped strength and made for a hopeless despair at times which was never part of my former life. Considering the fact that I had normally worked more than one job, had stayed busy seven days a week writing or teaching, or working about the yard and house, and now was listless and suffering periodic bouts of almost complete apathy, it became clear early that something more serious was wrong. During one of those severe periods, when apathy was deepest, a misunderstanding with my spouse triggered off a divorce after thirty years of marriage and ten children.

Since there seemed to be a medically defined distinction between rheumatoid arthritis and degenerative arthritis — I was told (wrongly) that the former required considerable more rest and the second required active exercise of a moderate nature —I undertook to begin learning to play the piano and to also dance.

There's little question that the various physical exercises kept my joints fluid, although painfully so at times, but the greatest puzzle was in the fact that within two years of the initial diagnosis of "degenerative" arthritis, the small finger on the right hand began to turn sidewise, and a typical rheumatoid arthritis and hard nodule had begun to form at this joint. [Professor Roger Wyburn-Mason considered that all forms of arthritis should be rested, as joint activity increases inflammation and pain and prevents healing.]

Pains Increase

Pains continued to increase at various joints, and finally, about three years into the disease, my hands began to flush red and hot and to swell, especially on arising early mornings. A great number of like symptoms lasted throughout the day.

It became almost impossible for me to type on my regular manual typewriter, because of pain at the joints.

Now the little finger on the left hand began to twist also, and all the joints at the hands began to almost glow a firey red.

I was having difficulty opening ordinary bottles; catchup, pickle jars, soft drink; and the problem of opening small sacks of peanuts became a procedure of first cutting the celluloid wrappings wth a knife, instead of gripping and tearing with the fingers.

Lifting pots and pans became an exceedingly painful chore. Changing a tire without help was excruciatingly difficult.

My children could not understand why my habits had changed so drastically. Once there was nothing I would ask them to do in the way of farm or house maintenance that I would not chip in to do, also.

My spirit of hopelessness extended from myself to family to friends, and finally even to passing acquaintances who could instinctively sense the unhappiness carried about by a rapidly aging man.

How could one make fast friends when daily my body was changing, and daily I became weaker and much more ineffective with everything touched?

How could long-range committments be kept, or strong personal relations be acknowledged? How fair is it to impose on those you love such burdens: future helplessness and twisted grotesqueness?

I was sufficiently imaginative to know where it would end, and frankly did not want to burden anyone with what was coming. I would rather be dead than crippled and helpless and apathetic and daily sapping the youth and vitality of my children.

Still, having had an extensive scientific background (mathematics, chemistry, physics, psychology) and also a very wide-ranging background in many different disciplines, I started searching through technical literature (just as did Dr. Blount) and talking to people. Only by fortuitous accident did I come to be helped by Dr. Jack M. Blount, and it came about through this series of connections:

The Discovery

A daughter-in-law knew of my terrible pains and my search in the literature. She mentioned my search to parents. They had a friend who'd been to Dr. Blount and had been cured. They suggested to my daughter-in-law that her father-in-law write to Dr. Blount.

Like so many others in like predicament, I sent out the letter, not with great anticipation — frankly I thought I'd be fluffed off to my family doctor — but because by now (as those with the same condition know) one cannot afford to overlook anything.

Lo! A most amazing answer came back, consisting of three pages, that described Dr. Blount's own search and cure, as told in the preceding, and in that correspondence, without cost, was embedded the name and amount of the drug necessary to produce the cure.

The Cure

When I tried Dr. Blount's treatment, which lasted six weeks, here's what happened:

• After two weeks the puffiness and redness of fingers disappeared for the first time in a half year.

•   After four weeks the pain, depression and fatigue ended.

• After seven weeks the redness of finger joints nearly disappeared.

•   After seven weeks my attitude toward life and people changed remarkably, and again I felt that life was worth the effort, and so were people and personal relations.

There were still problems. The twisted little fingers are still distorted. Damaged, fused joints may never heal, but where capillaries exist, over time, healing may again proceed faster than self-destruction. There is some redness of the other finger joints from time to time, expecially when used for long periods at the typewriter. There was still some pain of other joints here and there. Dr. Blount said that experience shows most of these residual pains would settle out in time.

But, I was able daily to turn more bottle tops, and lift heavier loads, and wrestle playfully with another without screaming bloody murder!

And, best of all, extreme apathy was gone, as was middle-of-day fatigue!

Can there be a better gift from one human to another, than this, that health and happiness is restored, and at no cost, except that of minor medicines?

Need the author state: I loved Dr. Jack Blount and Professor Roger Wyburn-Mason, the first for courage, fortitude and charity, the second for wisdom, persistence and intelligence!

What has happened to
Anthony di Fabio since the above was written?

But there is more to getting and staying well than a couple of pills! In the search for a better quality of life since that date, I delved deeper into alternative therapies, knowing that traditional medical practices were futile.

To recap: A 57-year-old-male (now, 2015, 90), with stress from his job, marriage, and finances, had developed progressively increasing symptoms of heated and swollen joints. I had been filled with pain, lethargy and depression, and I often woke up nights finding my bed soaked with sweat. I was told by my family doctor that I had Rheumatoid Arthritis, that I would be crippled soon, and that there was no hope for me, other than the temporary easing of pain and other symptoms by means of Non-Steroidal Anti-inflammatory drugs (NSAIDS); and later, as the disease progressed, use of cortisone, gold shots and then methotrexate. (Rheumatologists now seem to reverse this progression, starting first with severely damaging methotrexate.)

The idea of being crippled was perhaps the greater fear, and even deeper lethargy and depression had set in.

Intuitively I knew that I had to relieve stress, and so I took necessary, painful, steps to do so. There was also a sufficient spark of hope in me to continue to search for alternatives, and at last, after trying various homefolk remedies proferred by one friend or another, I found the described treatment recommended by Roger Wyburn-Mason, M.D., Ph.D. and Jack M. Blount, M.D.

Dr. Blount, himself a victim of crippling Rheumatoid Arthritis for many years, sympathetically had taught me what do do, and which prescription medicines to take. Dr. Blount wrote prescriptions for metronidazole and allopurinol which I had taken, although my family doctor felt it would be safe but useless.

Within three days a severe Herxheimer effect[5] occurred -- a temporary intensification of the disease symptoms — and, had I not been strongly warned of these consequences of taking these prescription medicines, I would have assumed that my Rheumatoid Arthritis was now flaring up in an extreme manner -- getting worse than ever. More joints than before begin aching excrutiatingly, night sweats increased in severity, joints became more swollen and heated, and lethargy and depression had reached what I describe as "the pits."

The Herxheimer effect tapered off during the next six weeks. It became clear that all the key characteristics of Rheumatoid Arthritis were gone: pyrexia (heat), edema (swelling), lethargy and depression, night sweats and an increasing number of painful joints.

There had been a great deal of damage to me during the period that Rheumatoid Disease was progressing, and so various joints still held pain.

Dr. Paul Pybus, developer of Professor Roger Wyburn-Mason's Intra-Neural Injections[6] visited America from Africa and between Dr. Pybus and Gus J. Prosch, Jr., M.D. (who learned, extended, and taught Pybus'/Wyburn-Mason's technique), I began receiving intra-neurals every three to four months. The doctor would palpate — touch with his finger — key nerve ganglia near the surface of the skin. As these nerve ganglia led to joints with pain, whenever one was found with disturbed cellular nerve cell membranes, the doctor would mark the spot, and then inject it with a combination of Depot Medrol and a very dilute solution of Triamcinolone Hexacetonide, a pain killer and cellular membrane stabilizer. This combination of medicines, acting locally, not systemically, caused the pain in the joints to disappear immediately. Pybus' past evidence showed that such relief lasted anywhere from three months on up to five years. Over a period of two years, treatments taken three to six months apart, I observed that there were increasingly less painful nerve ganglia, and that the beneficial effects of the treatments lasted longer each time taken.

Also, every three to six months I had to repeat the prescription medicines, each time going through the Herxheimer effect, but not in the severe form first encountered, each Herxheimer lasted but a night, or at most, two nights.

After two years of this, I at last heeded Dr. Gus Prosch's[7] (and other physicians) advice to pay attention to diet and vitamin and mineral supplements, including avoiding the wrong kind of fats and oils, and consuming the correct kind of essential fatty acids. I began to change lifestyle based on the saliva litmus test designed by Carl Reich, M.D., finding that my saliva invariably gave an extremely pale "Ph" color indicating extreme acidic condition.

However, it was difficult for me to change life style, as 59 years (by now) of education in faulty nutritional advice had led me to live on fast food hamburgers, candy bars and pop, canned goods, margarine and so on.

As an experiment I studied the use of mega-dosages of vitamins and minerals, as described by Durk Pearson and Sandy Shaw[21] and grudgingly started eating fresh fruits, vegetables, whole grains and fresh-water fish. I also changed cooking oils to that of Virgin Olive Oil, and I used butter rather than margarine, supplemented with a quality grade of Flaxseed Oil, and I ate more nuts, such as walnuts, all according to Dr. Gus J. Prosch's advice.

While it took time to observe a difference, it eventually became clear that I no longer needed the intra-neural injections.

While the struggle to change diet continued, I still suffered from extreme tiredness and claudication in the legs, a pronounced symptom of pain and cramping on lying down. I learned of EDTA (Ethylene Diamine Tetracetic Acid) Chelation Therapy[8], and also DMSO (Dimethylsulfoxide) Intravenous (IV) Therapy[9], taking more than ninety five of the former and nine of the latter, although sometimes EDTA and DMSO were mixed together. It's clear from loss of specific symptoms, lab tests and ease of exercise that I benefited greatly from these intravenous (IV) treatments.

I also tried oral Hydrogen Peroxide[10] treatment, but could not tolerate the oral administration which produced in me extreme nausea. Later I had nine intravenous hydrogen peroxide treatments, which safely knocked out a long-standing infection.

I learned that all Rheumatoid Disease victims suffer from Candidiasis by reason of having had a weakened immunological system, and so I sought advice and treatment against these organisms-of-opportunity, also learning to supplement with *Lactobaccilus acidolphilus* and *Bifido bacterium[11]*, along with other vitamin, mineral and essential fatty acid supplements[12].

I found myself impotent, and after several trials and studies I twice injected bis-beta carboxyethyl germanium sesquioxide, Ge, which solved the impotency problem[13], but not wholly. Later, a combination of percutaneous (skin applied) mixture of DHEA (dehydroepiandrosterone) and testosterone completely solved the problem.

I successfully used the "five-day pure water diet," followed by single food challenges. This solved some difficult problems by permitting the body to detoxify, while also learning to which foods I was especially allergic.

Damage done to my body had resulted in extreme pain in the neck and shoulder, increasing in severity over a period of one year, which normally would have required spinal fusions. Fortunately, I discovered reconstructive therapy (sclerotherapy or proliferative therapy)[14] through William J. Faber, D.O. Dr. Faber referred me to James O. Carlson, D.O., who specialized in non-surgical sports medicine. Over the period of twelve months, one treatment per month, Dr. Carlson helped me restore my body's structure, pain-free. It should not have taken more than three to six months, but my basal metabolism was low. This I learned by the use of the Broda O. Barnes', M.D. armpit temperature measurement technique, and I was placed on thyroid replacement therapy for a period of time. As use of reconstructive therapy depends on the body's ability to repair itself, the basal metabolism must be functioning effectively for rapid success[15]. The work of E. Denis Wilson, M.D.[22] in defining and treating multiple enzyme deficiencies resulting from thyroid deficiencies provided a more permanent change in thyroid deficiency problems.

I completed a series of Rolfing massages, restoring my structural integrity, and also reducing a great deal of pain in the left leg, still leaving tendonitis from instability aggravated by fast (swing, jitterbug and country and western) dancing, which I still did to age of 82, three or four times per week. Chiropractice manipulation at last totally relieved residual foot pain.

For a period I suffered from active gout, and took for several years Colbenamid^{TM} (probenecid and colchicine)

and allopurinol. How it finally resolved itself is unknown[16].

I received live-cell therapy from Lester Winter, Ph.D. and found some improvement in a skin condition and in hypoglycemia. Later, to solve a roughened up meniscus on my right knee, I received live-cell therapy from Hector Solorzano del Rio, M.D., Ph.D., D.Sc., Guadalajara, Mexico.

From Susana Alcazar Leyva, M.D. I received injections of a form of thiamine (cocarboxylase) and nicotinamide dinucleotide plus adenine. These self-administered shots, taken twice weekly, greatly improved energy through, presumably, improvement of metabolic activity. Again, unfortunately, I've not been able to complete her treatment.

My tendonitis problem was intransigent for more than four years, and calcium spurs were beginning to interfere with my ability to type. I therefore began exploring new means to resolve these two problems. [The tendonitis seems to be resolved by use of ELF Works, Inc. (St. Francisville, ILL) Light Beam Generator[19].

Despite bothersome Osteoarthritis and calcium spurs — for which I'm searching for answers —I can report a renewed lease on life — at least my quality of life —I want everyone to know what I've accomplished.

I also want folks to know that I've still got other problems stemming from prior damage done by the raging disease process, and also aging problems, accompanied with some long time mold and house-dust allergy problems. I follow my own advice, by searching out means for solving, not just alleviating, symptoms[65].

I will probably investigate one thing or another until the day my whole system finally gives out, probably like the one-hoss shay, all at once.

One thing is clear: Rheumatoid Disease is a great crippler unless the individual is willing to search out and to use treatment modalities that are not otherwise accepted by the established medical doctrines; and further, that the patient be willing to take personal responsibility for his/ her own recovery, not despairing because one doctor or one form of treatment is not successful, but rather going on to find the one suited to one's own unique condition.

The above case history is presented to demonstrate what can be done if you're determined to get well, and to improve the quality of your livingess.

References

1. *Modern Medicine*, "Rheumatoid Disease: Has One Investigator Found Its Cause and Its Cure?" Robert Bingham, M.D., Feb. 15, 1976, pp. 38-47.

2. *The Causation of Rheumatoid Disease and Many Human Cancers*, Roger Wyburn-Mason, M.D., Ph.D., Iji

Publishing Co, Ltd., Japan.. Out of print; Wyburn-Mason's *Addenda* (pre'cis and summary) is available from Kindle and Nook.

3. Joan Wyburn-Mason, *Dedication, Love and* Op.Cit., 1985 available on Kindle and Nook.

4. Jack M. Blount, M.D., Archimedes Concon, M.D., James Rowland, D.O.,William Renforth, M.D., Paul Williamson, M.D., Roger Wyburn-Mason, M.D., Ph.D., *Historical Documents In Search of the Cure for Rheumatoid Disease,* www.arthritistrust.org; Op.Cit., 1985.

5. Dr. Paul K. Pybus, *The Herxheimer Effect,* www.arthritistrust.org; Op.Cit., 1992.

6. Dr. Paul K. Pybus, *Intraneural Injections for Rheumatoid Arthritis and Osteoarthritis,* 1989, and *The Control of Pain in Arthritis in the Knee,* at Kindle and Nook Op.Cit., 1984.

7. Gus J. Prosch, Jr., M.D., Anthony di Fabio, *Proper Nutrition for Rheumatoid Arthritis,* www.arthritistrust.org; Op. Cit. 1994.

8. Anthony di Fabio, *Chelation Therapy,*www.arthritistrust.org; Op. Cit. 1993.

9. Efrain Olszewer, M.D., Fuad C. Sabbag, M.D., Alan Rory Zapata, M.D. *DMSO (Dimethylsulfoxide) Treatments in Arthritis,* www.arthritistrust.org, Op.Cit., 1994.

10. Charles H. Farr, M.D., Ph.D., *Hydrogen Peroxide Therapy,* www.arthritistrust.org, Op. Cit. 1989.

11. Anthony di Fabio, *Friendly Bacteria - Lactobaccilus acidophilus & Bifido bacterium,*www.arthritistrust.org, Op. Cit. 1989.

34

12. Gus J. Prosch, Jr., M.D./Anthony di Fabio, *Essential Fatty Acids are Essential*, www.arthritistrust.org, Op. Cit., 1989.

13. Anthony di Fabio, *Germanium* , www.arthritistrust.org, Op. Cit., 1989.

14. Morton J. Walker, D.P.M., William J. Faber, D.O., James Carlson,D.O./Anthony di Fabio, *Treatment of First Choice for Osteoarthritis and Other Arthritic-Like Pain: Sclerotherapy, Proliferative Therapy, Reconstructive Therapy*; www.arthritistrust.org, Op.Cit. 1994; also see *Pain, Pain Go Away* by Morton Walker, D.P.M., William J.Faber, D.O.

15. Anthony di Fabio/Broda Barnes, M.D., *The Master Regulator: Thyroid Therapy*, www.arthritistrust.org, Op. Cit., 1989.

16. John Baron, D.O., *Gouty Arthritis* , www.arthritistrust.org, Op. Cit., 1989.

17. Anthony di Fabio, *Rheumatoid Diseases Cured at Last*, Kindle or Nook, also many bookstores for online books, Op. Cit., 1982.

18. Durk Pearson and Sandy Shaw, *Life Extension*, Warner Books, inc., 666 Fifth avenue, New York,10103, June 1983.

19. Thomas Gervais, Courtland Reeves, Anthony di Fabio, *Lymphatic Detoxification*, www.arthritistrust.org, Op.Cit., 1994.

20. Royden Brown, *Bee Pollen: The Perfect Food,* www.arthritistrust.org, Op.Cit., 1994.

21. Durk Pearson, Sandy Shaw, *Life Extension*, Warner Books, Inc., 666 Fifth Avenue, New York, NY 10103, 1983.

22. E. Denis Wilson, M.D., *Wilson's Syndrome*, Cornerstone Publishing Company, 4524 Curry Ford Road, Suite 211, Orlando, FL 32812, 1993.

For all those paragraphs not footnoted, see other publications of The Rheumatoid Disease Foundation.

Arthritics' Primary Treatment Protocol
Can Rheumatoid Arthritis Be Cured? You've been told that Rheumatoid Arthritis is not curable. That is false!

If the statement disturbs you, do not read further. Do not learn how thousands are finding relief and even wellness. Do not give up your aspirin, your non-steroidal anti-inflammatories. Do not quit your visits to your favorite rheumatologist. Do not stop paying for ineffective and damaging gold, penicillamine, methotrexate and cortisone.

On the other hand, if you're among those who are filled with pain day and night, and want relief — if you're a person who views the future as a cripple with constantly decreasing abilities and want to stop the crippling — if you're a man or woman or child who lives pain-free but minutes and then only at the will of a drug, a doctor, a drug store, and by courtesy of a fat pocketbook — but especially if you're a person who wants relief from this centuries-long scourge — you'll want to absorb all of our literature in its entirety -and you'll want to read further!

At least thirteen million Americans suffer from so-called incurable Rheumatoid Diseases. Three million are restricted in their daily activities. Seven hundred thousand cannot do useful work, keep house, attend school or enjoy recreational activities. One out of three of us either have a form of the disease or will display some symptoms
— if we live long enough!

Tens o f millions o f Americans suffer from Osteoarthritis and Gouty Arthritis. Some predict that almost everyone will develop some form of Arthritis if she/he lives long enough.

Incidentally, we take the stand that there is no difference in causation between so-called "Adult Rheumatoid Arthritis" and "Juvenile Rheumatoid Arthritis." Both age groups respond to the treatments to be described.

If left untreated, Rheumatoid Arthritis and other forms of collagen tissue diseases [Rheumatoid Diseases] can become progressively worse, eventually leading to painful crippling, but this is particularly true of Rheumatoid Arthritis, which can and will destroy the joints unless effective treatment is administered in time.

Those who tell you that nothing much can be done for Arthritis are only fooling themselves and you. A great deal can be done, as you will learn — and crippling is not inevitable.

Most arthritis victims suffer pain, but we can show several ways that pain can be controlled and possibly alleviated entirely.

The sooner you begin treatment for Arthritis, the more probability of having success in halting its progress and perhaps cleaning up or reversing damage that has begun.

When there are those who tell you that, "Once you have Arthritis, chances are great that you're stuck with it for life," and "You should learn to adjust to it, for better or worse." "Don't look for a cure or relief, but learn to control your symptoms" — those people are telling you to give up, to permit the crippling to go on, to get yourself ready for a life of total misery and acceptance of your fate.

Those same advisors are also ignorant of any other means of helping you, or they would not be giving you such advice. They have given up. You don't need to give up too!

You must make a choice. Do you wish to follow such do-nothing-but-damage "establishment" medical practices? Or do you wish to fight for your survival and some of the good things in life, including the right to live unhindered from pain and crippling?

No pharmaceutical company is interested in curing or stopping the progress of our disease. They are interested in maintaining our dependency drug habits so that corporate stock owners and upper management can swell up their pocketbooks. Ideally, when a drug company can develop an exclusive, patented drug upon which arthritics must rely — as a drug addict must rely on habit-forming drugs — then the drug company is content. They are especially happy if the medicine relieves symptoms and forces us to spend more and more on the drug to simply maintain the appearance of wellness — and the disease rages onward!

The House subcommittee on health and the environment (1987) investigated hikes in prescription-drug prices — a 12.2 percent increase between July 1985 and April 1987 (versus only a 2.7 percent increase in the Consumer Price Index during that time).

The subcommittee staff obtained revenue data from the nation's 25 largest drug companies and prepared a report. Subcommittee chairman Henry Waxman summarized the findings at a hearing, saying, "Most of the money generated by the recent enormous price increases is not going to fund Research & Development. Between the years 1982 and 1986, drug price increases produced revenue gains of $4.7 billion. During the same period, Research & Development expenditures rose only

$1.6 billion — or about a third of the revenue gains from price increases.

"In short, the money was arriving in bucketloads, but was going to Research & Development in spoonfuls," Waxman said.

Apparently Waxman did not understand that drug companies are not interested in achieving wellness!

Cortisone provides only symptomatic relief, as its sale and medicinal administration to arthritics illustrates very well. Cortisone provides temporary and spectacular pain relief and the glow of false wellness. We must take increasing quantities over time to achieve this effect at the level we received earlier. During that period our bodies produce less and less of it. Eventually, over time, we quit producing cortisol at all. (Hydrocortisone: closely related to cortisone.) Thereafter, over time, we're hooked, and without periodic cortisone purchased from a drug company, by doctor's prescription, we die.

Our recommended treatments may not restore your ability to produce your own cortisol, a substance similar to cortisone, and it may not restore your deformed joints, but read on. It may restore your hope in a livable future, a sense of adventure, and a faith that you've possibly buried beneath tons of pain and agony. It may restore wellness!

Treated by the hundreds of physicians who follow our treatment protocol properly, there are already tens of thousands of former arthritics — folks like you and me — who have found great relief, improvement and yes, even complete wellness.

I was an arthritic — perhaps just as you are now — but I am free of the horrible disease and have been for 23 years.

I intend to convince you to take command of your life again, to learn for yourself ways and means of achieving wellness and again peace of mind. I will describe what you can do, recommend books to read, and that you work with a caring physician. If necessary, you must search out and find a physician who is not bound by that ancient arrogance which prevents some physicians from learning further and the patient from achieving wellness.

Eighty percent of those who follow my directions will either be cured or improved immensely and the disease halted. If you are among those whose bodily functions (immunological system) have already been damaged by traditional treatments that use gold, penicillamine, methotrexate and long-term cortico-steroids, the news is still favorable and better than your present outlook. About 50% of this latter group get well or vastly improved, especially when they are willing and able to halt these destructive treatments for four months prior to starting the one recommended herein. Usually after permitting bodily systems to recover throughout four months, the immunological system responds sufficiently to our treatment.

Traditional treatment can expect to achieve relief or the temporary appearance of wellness but 33% of the time. The placebo effect — the percentage of patients who will improve (at least temporarily) no matter what the physician does — is about 33% for arthritics. It follows, therefore, that traditional treatments are not effective any better than chance alone, and for that dubious privilege of non-wellness we pay out $15 billion a year.

The treatments described in this article are therefore at least 165% better than traditional, accepted but ineffective treatments.

Niether I or The Arthritis Trust of America have vested interests in the sale of drugs, foods, medical treatments, vitamins and minerals, physicians or clinics. I work for a non-profit, charitable, tax-exempt foundation dedicated to solving the problems of Arthritis by means of education and research.

This article tells how Dr. Jack M. Blount and I got well from this horrible scourge and at the end of this book it condenses our findings since 1982, and while our recommendations are in advance of anything else written on arthritis, it will not be the last and final word. Scientific progress means change. Solving Rheumatoid Arthritis and related diseases means changing both the modalities of present-day treatment and our own attitudes toward it.

To your family doctor, we say: Our treatment protocol has never been considered for use against Rheumatoid Arthritis because the various rheumatologists and arthritis associations have not investigated Professor Roger

Wyburn-Mason's brilliant scientific work, published since

1964 that led to the treatment to be described. Neither have they conducted proper scientific studies to demonstrate the importance of nutritional factors, Candidiasis and food allergies on collagen tissue diseases.

You must, therefore, decide if the prescriptions and treatment recommendations that follow are harmful to your patient. If not, is the cost involved worth a trial, considering the hopeless and insidious nature of the disease?

Many cooperating physicians, and their patients, use and have used the protocol — more than two hundred physicians, tens of thousands of patients, represented in many countries.

Our referral physicians contributed greatly to this book through their clinical experiences.

We cannot, of course, be responsible for mal-application, misapplication, or inappropriate treatment of any kind, and suggest strongly that treatment, if possible, be through your family physician or through an open minded physician.

I pray that you will be among those who read and follow recommendations where appropriate.

Our common goal?

To rid the earth of this terrible, crippling plague, called Arthritis!

You Must Judge

An arthritic needs no description of his disease's progress, nor his painful symptoms that distort the joints into such grotesque forms, leading inevitably to surgery and certain crippling. But even the arthritic needs to be able to differentiate those arthritic symptoms that represent an on-going disease process — active disease — as compared to the damage that has already been done or will be done.

Symptoms of an active, on-going disease process are usually tissue swelling (edema), warm or hot joints (pyrexia), lethargy and depression, night sweats, and, most importantly, an increasing number of painful joints.

When we state that we can stop the progress of Rheumatoid Disease for 80% of the victims who properly use our treatment protocol, we speak specifically of halting and reducing tissue swelling, halting night sweats, restoring joints and tissues to normal temperature and stopping the <u>increase</u> in the number of joints that become affected and painful. Depression and lethargy may also stop, and will certainly do so with further related treatments of a different nature, as might also be required for the pain that may remain in joints after wellness is restored. It is totally possible, and has happened frequently, that no related treatments will be required, but don't count on a simple approach to clear up everything at once.

So what about the already crippled-up joints, and residual pain and lethargy and depression that might remain The on-going disease process reflects itself through

the swelling (edema) and heat (pyrexia), and just as these are symptomatic processes — evidence that something is wrong — the <u>result</u> of all those biochemical processes shows up as damaged, painful joints, lethargy and depression.

There is more complexity, but we shall unwind a lot of it. For now, remember the term "free-radical damage." For the purpose of this book, we shall define "free-radical damage" as secondary damage that accompanies Rheumatoid Disease while it is active or "flared up." This definition is not scientifically accurate or complete, but neither is this a manuscript of science.

Even if you are an arthritic, you have probably been viewing your symptoms in a way that includes <u>all</u> characteristics of the disease — the "on-going process" characteristics and the "secondary damage" characteristics caused by the "on-going process" — as a complete package. How many times have you seen or heard the comment, "Oh, that's Rheumatoid Disease" when speaking of a crippled joint?

No!

The crippled joint is not the disease!

The crippled joint is a result of the disease!

When our treatment is used, and when it is effective, the symptoms of swelling and heated joints disappear, and the symptoms of joint pain may disappear, as may the symptoms of lethargy and depression. Most certainly other treatments to be described will probably rid one of left over joint pains and lethargy and depression unless irreversible damage is involved, such as permanently deformed joints. I have two small fingers with permanently deformed joints, for example; but no longer do I have Rheumatoid Arthritis.

Reporting on many case histories are nice, and emotionally convincing to the layman, but they do absolutely nothing to convince scientists and physicians, who require different proof forms. University medical research as funded by you and others will satisfy them, not this book, nor any number of case histories. Even if success stories number in the tens of thousands as our referral physicians can already describe, medical scientists remain unconvinced. You have probably tried many other treatments that have not worked, and you will not be fearful of trying one more. You, like me, are probably tired of reading case histories of alleged success. Our treatment either works on you, or doesn't work at all. You and I care less about whether it worked on others, until we solve our own problem.

Like you, I was skeptical and even scoffed — but I tried these recommended treatments, for lack of anything better.

Even my family doctor scoffed, saying, "Look, it won't help, but it can't harm you, so go ahead and try if you wish," and with that he unknowingly started me on the path to wellness.

The truth is — and so it is true of the scientific method — that no number of hearsay statements from and about successful patients will answer your big question. Since the treatment is safe under proper medical supervision — extremely safe when compared against traditional treatments — your only question is, "will it be effective for me?" There is no way to answer such a question without giving our treatment protocol a fair trial — and only you will know whether or not you have tried honestly and fairly.

Be forewarned that many of the treatment methods to be described for you are not accepted treatments. Some related treatments to be described and which have also proved effective are being persecuted by unknowledgeable state medical boards and duped district attorneys in some states. While this blind rejection is not true of everything to be described, by being forewarned you will be able to better cope with scoffers and authoritarian figures who feel their control — and income — slipping away.

If Authorities knew the correct treatment, they would already be applying it, wouldn't they?

So don't be embarrassed if some would-be larger than life Authority denounces what is said herein, or argues against your trial of various treatments. Progress in medicine has always been thusly hindered, and your job as a patient is to separate the "It works for me!" from "It doesn't work for me!" And no number of Authorities can make it otherwise, and no one knows better than you whether or not the treatment fits one category or another.

Our recommendations to get you well are for the most part safe, effective and cheap.

Remember this!

Not all the Authorities on earth and their scholastic, little, hobgoblined opinions can determine whether or not our treatment works for you!

You must judge for yourself!

Rheumatoid Disease Newly Defined

The human body has a limited number of responses to various system disturbances. For example: Most everyone is familiar with headaches. While the pain of each headache may be very similar in nature each time experienced, the cause of each headache can vary considerably. Headaches might be caused by eyestrain, back or low musculature strain, biological disturbances of tissues or chemistry, suppressed emotion, and so on.

In other words, just because a person has a headache does not mean that the cause is self-evident, or necessarily simple, nor does the cause of our headache need to be related to the causes of our neighbors or friends.

While we are all genetically different, and have different biochemistries, our bodies seem to have limited ways of responding to varying stimuli.

It should be clear, therefore, that all symptoms described as "arthritic" are not symptoms that derive from the same cause. You probably already know about "Osteoarthritis," "Rheumatoid Arthritis" and "Gouty Arthritis," three of the most common with differing causes.

Rheumatoid Arthritis is characterized by specific symptoms: heated joints and body members, swelling, lethargy, depression and an increasing number of painful joints that eventually become damaged and crippled.

Since we look at only symptoms of a disease "in-process" we cannot say for sure that every time someone has these five characteristics he/ she has the same disease cause as others.

When laboratory tests are used to narrow the causative agent(s), we are often led to costly tests that are virtually useless. The test that is labeled "RF" for "Rheumatoid Factor" is mis-labeled and probably does not test for Rheumatoid Arthritis at all. It tests a fraction of blood called "immunoglobulin" and is present in 70% of adults with Rheumatoid Arthritis. Some physicians have indicated that 25% of such tests are negative, when they should be positive, and 25% are positive when they should be negative. At best, the test measures probable existence of something akilter respecting our bodily systems, a fact we already know.

It is highly unlikely that any number of present-day laboratory tests (1996) can determine the existence or non-existence of Rheumatoid Disease. Often the physician makes such tests because it is the established and accepted thing to do, and because doing the established and accepted thing protects his/her medical insurance and medical license status. Neither of these reasons gets you properly diagnosed or well.

Sometimes these lab tests together with clinical experience and good judgment can deduce a set of possible causes that should be further explored by medical treatment trials. Those trials, even if unsuccessful, may lead to further educated guesses on the part of your physician that will eventually narrow causes down to one or more that are amendable to changes.

Your problem may be to find a physician who is willing to step outside of traditional treatment boundaries and to view you as a whole person, not just a statistic to warehouse in a small examination room pending arrival of his august presence, and there to be scrutinized but minutes, and thereafter to be given at relatively high cost a traditional, accepted, ineffective treatment.

Many in the medical community suspect a causative organism for Rheumatoid Disease such as bacteria, mycoplasma, yeast/fungus, protozoan, virus, cell wall deficient organism, or some combination or variation of these minute life forms.

They suspect that people are either born with a genetic susceptibility to these organisms or develop that genetic susceptibility later. "Genetic susceptibility" means an inborn sensitivity to the organism or toxin from the organism that causes our tissues to respond with the symptoms of "arthritis."

There is a high degree of suspicion that we have developed, or are born with, an "allergy" to some organism that invades from outside our bodies. We develop "antibodies," fighters, for that "antigen," the invader, and there comes persistent warfare between our antibodies and the antigen that creates damage we see as the symptoms we call Rheumatoid Disease.

This suspicion may very well be based on truth, and it serves as a good model, really the best predictor and hypothesis of the nature of the disease that we have to date. From a purely workable viewpoint, we can accept the model until developing a better one.

The antibody/antigen model serves to underline one very important aspect of Rheumatoid Disease. The disease is not localized in just one place! The disease is systemic. This means that even though you do not observe symptoms of the disease as raging onward in a particular portion of your body -- as when you're under the influence of cortisone — the disease is there, actually everywhere, believe me.

It may be for the moment you are manifesting the disease in a particular part of the body. These overt symptoms make you think the disease is localized to, say, a knee joint, or wrist joint. All of your attention is quite naturally on that spot, because that's where the pain, swelling and heat is for the moment.

If you accept the proposition that Rheumatoid Disease is systemic (throughout the body) in nature, it is clear that a treatment for purely local parts of the body is doomed to failure. Cortisone shots to relieve pain in a joint, for example, do not stop the process in either the joint or in the whole body, while they do help to erode the joint further.

There are two characteristics about Rheumatoid Disease to keep in mind. One is that Rheumatoid Disease symptoms may be the result of multiple causes. We see similarities between different people because our bodies are designed to respond in but limited ways. The second fact is that Rheumatoid Disease pervades the whole body, not just a local area.

Having stated the above two principles, we now mention possible "causes" of "arthritis."

The symptoms of "arthritis" may be "caused," that is, actually produced or mimiced, by any one or combination of the following:

1. Bacterial infections such as those resulting from invasion of gonococcal, tuberculosis, or pneumococcal germs.

2. Viruses, particularly RNA viral forms.

3. Yeast/fungus, particularly *Candida albicans*.

4. Allergens, internal and/or external, as with foods, pollens, house dusts, invading organisms.

5. Weakened immunological system, caused by any of the above and including causation of improper nutrition, prolonged stress, etc.

6. Metabolic disturbances, as evident with Gout, Osteoarthritis, Osteoarthrosis.

7. Other unidentified and unnamed source causes. All of the above, and perhaps more, may cause

symptoms of Rheumatoid Arthritis. The portions of the body where the symptoms may appear are a multitude. To name a few, they are:

The arteries, as in periarteritis; Bone, as in Paget's Disease, cysts and myelomas; Brain and Spinal Cord, as displayed by tremors and seizures; Bronchi, as with bronchitis, intrinsic asthma (as opposed to extrinsic; i.e. caused by an external allergen or external source); Heart, as with dysrhythmias, myocardial disease, pericardial disease; Cecum as with appendicitis, mesenteric adenitis; Colon, as with ulcerative colitis; Endocrine glands, as with thyroid, parathyroid, thymus, pituitary, adrenal glands; Esophagus and Stomach, producing atropic mucosa (pernicious anemia), webs; Eyes, with iridocyclitis, exophthalmias; fascial planes, showing as bursitis; Female Genitals, for ovarian cysts, fibroids, salpingitis-sterility, tubal pregnancies; Hemopoetic, displaying as Systemic Lupus Erythematosus, polycythemia, purpura; joints, as with arthritis; Kidneys, pyelonephritis, calculi; Liver, showing as hepatitis, cholangitis, gallbladder disease; Lower Small Gut, displaying as regional enteritis, Crohn's disease; Lungs as with alveolitis; Lymphatics (Lymph system) for lymphomas, splenomegaly; Meninges (covering around brain), producing headache, meningomas; Muscles with myositis; Nerves, trigeminal neuralgia; Nose and Throat, presenting as rhinitis, eustachian salpingitis, enlarged tonsils and adenoids; Ovum, producing fetal deformities and abortions; Pancreas with pancreatitis, maturity diabetes, noninsulin dependent diabetes; Salivary and Tear Glands with SICCA syndrome; Skin with psoriasis, alopecia, erythemas, urticaria; Spine, degenerated discs and low back syndrome; Tendons for tendonitis, ganglion; Upper Gut with Coealic disease; and also functional Central Nervous System problems producing neuroses, psychosis and senility.

Since different parts of the body are involved, the symptoms presented to the physician are given different names, but many of those described can now be classified under one heading, that of "Rheumatoid Disease." This is the definition given by Professor Roger WyburnMason, a brilliant research physician from England, now deceased, and whose treatment methods led to the first major improvements and cures.

There is a parallel, by analogy, between the old and generally accepted view of "Rheumatoid Arthritis" and that cluster of diseases which your Foundation now titles "Rheumatoid Disease." Before the discovery of the tubercle baccilus, the germ that causes tuberculosis, there were about 100 differently named symptoms that patients presented to their doctor. The fact that each symptom was given a unique name sometimes appeased the patient, but certainly did not get them well.

After discovery of the tubercle bacillus all of those

100 or so names collapsed under the heading of "TB of the bone," "TB of the lungs," "TB of the skin," and so on.

When I went to grade school (thirties) I was taught that everyone on earth was exposed to the TB germ, but that only a small number of people were genetically susceptible to the organism, thus coming down with TB. This may or may not have been true, but as a parallel analogy, and to produce a working hypothesis around which Rheumatoid Disease can be solved, the essentials appear to correspond. Rheumatoid Disease (hereafter often referred to as RD), has been given nearly a hundred different names; it now has but one, "Rheumatoid Disease" or "RD" and it seems to have a "genetic predisposition factor," i.e. people seem to be susceptible along genetic lines (inherited) to whatever causes the apparent antigen/ antibody relationship. All the named diseases have a commonality. They are "collagen tissue diseases."

All of the previously described diseases — and perhaps more — can occur in their pure forms, or in combinations with any of the other "labeled" diseases.

Naming a disease, as you know, does not get the person well any more so than treating a disease with the wrong medicine, or by the wrong treatment protocol. Most of the established and accepted treatments for RD are based on the presumption that there is something wrong with the immunological system, that portion of the body that fights off infection by recognizing a foreign protein as "not-me." If this presumption is wrong, there will be endless hours spent unraveling the complexity of the very obscure immunological system. There are, in fact, tons of books on this one subject, and it requires a highly trained specialist simply to understand details. It's sort of like being in the middle of a tangled woods and, rather than stepping out to understand the woods as a whole, one spends a lifetime learning about and studying each individual growth.

A perfect example of this "scientific" medical problem once existed with the lack of understanding of syphilis as a disease caused by an organism. Until the finding of the syphilis spirochete, the symptoms of syphilis presented to the research physician a perfect picture of an "auto-immune" disease; i.e., a disease wherein the immunological system fails to identify portions of the body as "self" and attacks the body as "non-self."

Now we know better that syphilis is a disease caused by an organism that comes from outside the body. It is not the consequence of a "failed" immunological system, except in the sense that those who live life styles that weaken the immunological system are at higher risk for becoming infected with any kind of pathogenic organism.

But consider the present day consequences to millions (and to organized society) if research physicians continued to insist that syphilis was a failure of the immunological system, an auto-immune disease, as all characteristics seemed to have indicated before discovery of the spirochete! Tens of millions, perhaps hundreds of millions of dollars would have been expended in studying the immunological system, and thousands of dangerous drugs would have been invented and tried without success to modify or otherwise change a supposedly defective immunological system — to no avail!

But that situation indeed seems to prevail today in the attempt to understand and otherwise control arthritis!

We have no proof that those who pursue the small seedlings within the forest of the very complex immunological system are not correct. But they also have no proof that our hypothesis and treatment is not correct. We must be fair both ways, and perhaps both sides have a component of truth.

You and I as arthritic victims care less what is believed or known, so long as we get well!

We shall take the assumption that there is a causative organism of origin or origins unknown. While the brilliant Professor Roger WyburnMason, M.D., Ph.D., along with protozoologist Vice-Admiral Stamm thought they had identified the source-cause to be a simple, ever-present, *Limax amoeba*, our later research was unable to verify their work. However, *some* organism must be involved, because Wyburn-Mason's treatment, based on his theory, works. And from that presumption, simply as a working hypothesis, we expect to show 80% of those who try our treatments that they can indeed become greatly improved or cured completely.

Finally, to all of those who have written to this Foundation or will write to ask a certain question, we have the same advice. Since there are no definitive tests, if you wish to know if your particular symptoms will respond to the treatment to be described, you can only answer this yourself, by trying our recommendations fairly and honestly under supervision of a caring physician.

May both God and your own good sense go with you in the next adventure!

Rheumatoid Disease Foundation Treatment Protocol

There are four general parts to recommended treatment protocol: (1) prescription drugs of a certain kind, called "anti-amoebic," (2) proper nutrition, (3) treatment against candidiasis and food allergies, and (4) other treatments appropriate to each individual. (We'll summarize everything we've learned about arthritis since 1982 at the end of this book.)

This Foundation's prescription treatment protocol must be administered by a licensed physician, usually a Medical Doctor or Doctor of Osteopathy, or any physician who can prescribe the medicines that are to be recommended.

The physician must determine whether or not your body is capable of handling (metabolizing) the various medicines without danger, and whether or not interaction between various medicines that you may be taking will be safe.

Your physician must also make a determination that you do not suffer from neurological disease, such as Multiple Sclerosis (MS). If you have MS and should take some of the medicines described, the progress of your MS may advance — which is obviously not what is desired.

In case that scares you, keep in mind that in the *Physician's Desk Reference*[1] (a collection of drug companies' package inserts) the use of some of our recommended medicines already carries warning against use by Multiple Sclerosis victims, and that all ethical physicians know or seek to know the *Physician's Desk Reference* before prescribing for a patient.

Medicines used for the treatment and remission or cure of Rheumatoid Arthritis and related collagen diseases now called "Rheumatoid Diseases" are the following:

1. Metronidazole
2. Clotrimazole
3. Tinidazole

4. Nimorazole

5. Ornidazole

6. Allopurinol

7. Furazolidone

8. Diiodohydroxyquinon

9. Rifampin

10. Potassium Para Amino Benzoate

11. Copper Ions

Not all of the above medicines will work for everyone, and usually one must start with a commonly accepted medicine or combination of medicines, and make a trial, which will be described.

The brilliant English professor and physician, Roger WyburnMason, Ph.D., M.D., (deceased) discovered use of all of the above except Metronidazole, whose use for Rheumatoid Arthritis was discovered by the Mississippi physician, Jack M. Blount, Jr., M.D. (deceased); Diiodohydroxyquinon, whose use for these purposes was discovered by Robert Bingham, M.D. (deceased) of California; and Seldon Nelson, D.O. (deceased) of Michigan developed the use of Copper ions.

Our treatment protocol, which was designed by a committee of physicians under the umbrella of our referral physicians, and subsequently modified through clinical findings, follows:

Why you must get off of traditional drugs.

If you are being treated with gold, penicillamine or methotrexate, then quit! Wait four months before taking our prescription treatment, as your immunological system has already been so upset by these ineffective and often damaging chemicals that your body probably will not respond well if at all to any of our medicines. DO NOT

TAKE OUR TREATMENT AT THE SAME TIME YOU ARE TAKING GOLD, PENICILLAMINE, METHOTREXATE OR ANY OTHER CYTOTOXIC DRUGS. GET OFF FROM CORTICOSTEROIDS, IF POSSIBLE. If you do take the above drugs simultaneously with our treatment, you are simply laying the groundwork for maintaining the disease and related diseases at the same time you are using our recommended medicines to rid yourself of the disease. The reason, to be described, is related to the weakening of your ability to fight diseases generally, the inability to repair yourself, and to the effects of severe drug toxicity when using traditional remedies.

****

The Effects of Cortisone

The effects of the use of corticosteroids (cortisone) are found at the microscopic level. It inhibits the early phenomena of the inflammatory process which includes swelling (edema), fibrin deposition (fibrin is responsible for blood clotting), capillary expansion (dilatation), migration of leukocytes (white blood cells) into the inflamed area, and phagocytic activity. Phagocytes search out and engulf and destroy foreign invaders. Cortisone also inhibits capillary proliferation, fibroblast proliferation, deposition of collagen and later scar tissue formation, all necessary for body growth and repair.

Cortisone has many well-known undesirable side-effects. It impairs wound healing and provides a predisposition to infection. It has major effects upon the monocyte/macrophage system, preventing release of Interleukin 1, a substance that aids in fighting diseases. Large doses of corticosteroids results in a secondary problem of lymphopenia, a deficiency of lymphocytes in the blood. Monocytes are large mononuclear (one nucleus) leukocytes having more protoplasm (a thick viscous colloidal substance which constitutes the basis of all living activities) than a lymphocyte. Lymphocytes are lymph cells or white blood corpuscles without cytoplasmic granules (cytoplasmic protoplasm of a cell outside the nucleus). Macrophages have the ability to phagocytose (absorb and destroy) substances. Among our first line of defense against foreign invaders are to be found lymphocytes and macrophages.

If the language disturbs you, do not be concerned. Just remember that in people receiving cortisone, monocytes (large leukocytes that kill invaders) show an impaired ability to kill microorganisms. In the test tube there is an inhibition in the proliferation of T cells. Helper and suppressor T cells in the blood stream have to be in the proper ratio, and they have a vital part in defending the body from foreign invaders. They also act in certain ways that causes macrophages to release the Interleukin 1. Interleukin 1 stimulates formation of Interleukin 2, the immediate stimulus for proliferation of T cells.

Corticosteroids (cortisone) lead to an increase in the number of polymorphonuclear leukocytes (white blood cells whose nucleus appear in different forms) in the blood. The lymphocytes, eosinophils (also a leukocyte but one that stains readily with an acid stain, eosin), monocytes and basophils (a type of leukocyte of heavy course granules which stain with basic dyes) decrease in number in the blood stream.

Corticosteroids interfere with a variety of functions, including intra-cellular killing, which is an anti-inflammatory effect. One common mechanism for anti-inflammatory effects is to enhance the production of a specific protein called "lipomodulin," which inhibits "phospholipase A[2]" which in turn is the enzyme necessary for the release of "arachidonic acid" from membrane phospholipids (fatty acid containing phosphorus). Arachidonic acid promotes the "arachidonic cascade" derived prostaglandins effects on cardiovascular, smooth muscle and has other effects. There then follows reduced synthesis of active metabolites (resulting products of the biochemical actions) of arachidonic acid. Arachidonic acid precedes the prostaglandins that result in the inflammatory phenomena. Aspirin and many other non-steroidal anti-inflammatories (NSAIDS) are aimed at inhibiting the production of prostaglandins, which then inhibits the inflammatory symptoms.

The results of all of the phenomena described with such technical medical words is seen mostly in the increased incidence of infection usually controlled by cellular immunity, which means an increase in infections of mycobacterial, fungal, nocardial and cytomegaloviral infections — bacteria, fungus, virus, etc. Obviously, if micro-organisms are the basis to Rheumatoid Disease — and they seem to be — then cortisone simply provides an easier route for more Rheumatoid Disease!

Steroids are also used widely in transplantations involving kidney, heart, liver, and bone marrow. In part, subsequent infections that are usually news-media-wise blamed on infections after transplantations is a direct result of use of the corticosteroids as well as other drugs.

Bacterial arthritis is an acute process that occurs in a joint following infection by any one of several microorganisms. Patients who receive intra-articular (in the joint) corticosteroids and those with existing Rheumatoid Arthritis appear to be predisposed to bacterial arthritis. Use of corticosteroids can stimulate and enhance this predisposition.

When corticosteroids result in increased susceptibility to various organisms, the list resembles the agents to which patients with Hodgkin's disease or acquired immune deficiency syndrome (AIDS) are vulnerable. Cryptococcal (fungus infection affecting any organ or tissue) infection is a rare infection overall, but at least half of all patients have some type of immune depression. Steroids can unmask latent Mycobacterium tuberculosis. Nocardial (gram positive bacteria) infections usually involving the lungs or brain occur in patients receiving long-term corticosteroids for a variety of indications (symptoms and signs) including Systemic Lupus Erythmatosus and organ transplantation. Listeria monocytogenes causes serious infection in infants who are otherwise healthy and in adults who are immunosuppressed by steroids or lymphreticular (lymph system) malignancy.

There are other negative effects from the use of corticosteroids, but the preceding list should be sufficient to explain why it is necessary to get off of this drug as quickly as possible, and also why the percentage of those helped by our treatment drops drastically when the patient uses some combination of gold, penicillamine, methotrexate, other cytotoxic drugs and long-term corticosteroids. While I have described the cortisone characteristics, gold, penicillamine and methotrexate, as will be seen, have even worse side-effects.

****

All of the traditional treatments affect the immunological system in various ways, and the list lengthens as more and more of these damaging medicines are used to suppress symptoms while permitting the disease to rage onward.

Decrease and Get Rid of Cortisone!

All of the forewarnings given were to say this: If you are hooked on cortisone, then start decreasing the dosage, under proper medical supervision. Decreasing the dosage of cortisone can be dangerous if you have reached a stage where daily or weekly shots or oral pills have replaced your body's natural ability to produce cortisol (your body's cortisone). Except for those people who no longer have any ability to produce cortisol for themselves, you MUST get off from any kind of cortisone, whether in the oral form of prednisone or given as injections, or purchased in Mexico under some brand name or through a clinic, or mixed with herbs of various vintage. Again there is another reason, that is, cortisone usage, while damping down symptoms, also permits Arthritis and related diseases to spread. Cortisone also interferes with the effectiveness of our treatment.

Non-Steroidal Anti-Inflammatory Drugs

If you are on aspirin, or aspirin substitutes called NSAIDS after the phrase "Non-steroidal Anti-Inflammatory Drugs" (indomethacin, phenylbutazone, etc.) then you may continue using any of these within safe limits. Their usage will not interfere with the treatments and may not cause your immunological system to weaken. When our treatments are completed successfully you should be pain free, or on minimum dosages of NSAIDS.

The Successful Treatment

In our treatment protocol, and on first trial, you should take simultaneously Metronidazole and Allopurinol. Based on a 170 pound weight, you should take 2 grams of Metronidazole either in one dosage, or distributed throughout four equal treatments, per day. You should take this dosage for two days in a row, then skip for five days.

You should repeat this procedure in all for six weeks. During the first week only, you should take 300 mg

of Allopurinol 3 times a day, for 7 days, then quit, taking only the Metronidazole throughout the remaining 5 weeks.

For each 25 pounds you weigh over or under 170 pounds, you should increase or decrease, respectively, your dosage of Metronidazole by 1/4 gram or 250 milligrams.

Five hundred milligram tablets are fine, but if your physician prescribes Metronidazole in 250 mg pills, then you can easily adjust the amount taken by your weight. For example, if you weigh 120 pounds, then you need to reduce the amount of Metronidazole taken by 1/2 gram, or two 250 mg tablets, because the difference between 170 pounds and 120 pounds is 50 pounds, which is two 25 pound units less than the treatment formula calls for a

170 pound person. Similarly, therefore, if you weigh 240 pounds, you need to increase the dosage to 2-1/2 grams. A child, therefore, can be administered proper dosage simply by observing the weight and subtracting accordingly. Approximations to the closest 25 pound unit is acceptable.

This technique of dosage by weight is common with prescription writing, because the human body's capability of metabolizing — converting chemicals and food to usable substances, or detoxifying poisons — is often directly correlated to weight.

It happens that all of the 5-nitroimidazoles (Metronidazole, Tinidazole, Clotrimazole, Ornidazole, Nimorazole) are chemically related where, in a five ring nitrogen structure molecule, the first nitrogen position (as defined by organic chemists) is replaced by another set of atoms or molecules. It also turned out that this is the only nitroimidazole nitrogen substitution that seems to be effective for arthritis without also causing damage. This doesn't mean that others will not be found, nor that some other compounds substituted in the first nitrogen position will not be dangerous. It does mean that so far as we know today, whenever a 5-nitroimidazole compound has the first of five nitrogen atoms replaced, and if the compound is also safe for human use, then it is probably effective for various Rheumatoid Diseases to some degree, and with many people.

Before describing what to expect after taking the above medicines, I will describe the remainder of our protocol, as the effects to be expected are similar in most instances.

Allopurinol should be taken with the 5-nitroimidazole the first week, at 300 mg 3 times per day, then terminated at the end of the seventh day.

If you are one of the rare people allergic to Allopurinol, your doctor may substitute Furazolidone in the following dosage: 100 mg, four times a day for one week only.

Either Allopurinol or Furazolidone may also be taken by themselves as may Metronidazole. However, if you are to benefit by our experiences, it is probably best to take the combination described as first trials. Together with one of the 5-nitroimidazoles, Allopurinol or Furazolidone are to help in providing broad spectrum anti-microrganism activity.

In the place of Metronidazole, one may take if available any of the other 5-nitroimidazoles, which includes Tinidazole, Clotrimazole, Nimorazole and Ornidazole. They may be taken in combination with Allopurinol or

Furazolidone, or by themselves. The dosage is exactly the same as described for Metronidazole, and the time period exactly the same.

Nimorazole and Ornidazole are available in some European countries, and perhaps elsewhere, but not in the United States. Tinidazole is easily available almost everywhere in the world. Tinidazole and Clotrimazole can be purchased in the United States and Canada from compounding pharmacists. Tinidazole is available at any drugstore in Mexico without a prescription under the trade names of Fasigyn or Tinidex.

Incidentally, the lower cost generic medicines in all of the drugs named are perfectly satisfactory.

Diiodohydroxyquinon (known as Iodoquinol) should be taken as 650 mg three times a day, for three weeks.

Potassium Para Amino Benzoate should be taken as 2 grams, 6 times daily for two weeks. This one is usually used for skin problems.

"Copper Ions" are small, resin granules upon which is deposited copper ions by a special process developed by Seldon Nelson, D.O. (deceased). Only five one-hundredths of a gram of copper per granule is deposited on each granule. These tiny granules are taken sub-lingually (beneath the tongue) in various ways: Usually the physician will start the patient with about 20 or 30 granules several times a day, increasing the amount by 10 or 20 per day, until a certain reaction is observed. Since large numbers of these small granules do not exceed the daily minimum requirement for copper, they do not require a prescription. Unfortunately, they cannot be easily obtained, as they were developed by Dr. Seldon Nelson for use with special patients.

Rifampin should be taken as 600 mg daily for one month. **Caution on use of this one, as it is a medicine that must be administered under close supervision, and if complications occur, then the physician should take you off of it immediately.**

If you have nausea with any of these medicines, your physician can prescribe an anti-nausea tablet.

I've just described all of the medicines and their dosages in our treatment protocol.

It is best to start with Metronidazole and Allopurinol if possible, but not necessary. It is best to use the various medicines individually or in the combinations already described, but not necessary. Usually most patients respond to the first medicines when used properly in the proper dosages, but there are a significant number that do not. One reason they do not has already been described: their past and possibly present use of gold, penicillamine, methotrexate (cytotoxic drugs) or long-term cortico-steroids. No one should deny such patients trials with our treatment for those reasons, but they should be made to understand (1) to get off of cortisone if at all possible and safe — and absolutely to get off of gold, penicillamine and methotrexate (cytotoxic drugs) for 4-months prior to our treatment; (2) that their response to our treatment may not be as sure, spectacular or swift as those not having been on such drugs; and (3) that they may need to use a number of other related and supporting treatments which, by the way, many others may also need in the long run, as is to be described.

Prior to taking Metronidazole, the physician should insure that the patient is provided with a good supplement of intestinal microflora, such as *Lactibacilus acidophilus*. Yogurt may or may not do as it is a bulgaris species. We have other objections to commercial Yogurt, as found in most supermarkets, in that they are often mixed with sugars and promote the growth of an arthritis-accompanying and   damaging organism called *Candida albicans*, a yeast fungus that can create similar symptoms to Arthritis, and other problems. I also object to the use of pasteurized products labeled as "acidophilus" this or that. If you kill the organisms by pasteurization, then why advertise their presence?

When you look around for a good grade of intestinal microflora supplement use caution. While it does not require a prescription to purchase *Lactibacilus acidophilus* from a health food store, you may be getting a poorly performing species, or, as bad, an organism that has already been weakened by environmental conditions. Any time temperature exceeds about 74 degrees Fahrenheit, the organism may lose viability or die, as when it is transported, left on the floor or in the stockroom of the   store   temporarily, or inadvertently placed   on nonrefrigerated shelves.

Physicians who administer this beneficial and symbiotic organism usually order from a company that is known to culture a good, viable grade, and who ship to you or your physician in protected containers.

Take about 1/4 teaspoon five or six times daily. Over about three weeks, you should begin to build up proper intestinal microflora so that these organisms will metabolize Metronidazole. Your enzyme system cannot do the job, and that helps to explain why Metronidazole does not always work with Rheumatoid Arthritics in   the dosages required. Metronidazole, being also anti-bacterial, may knock out "good guys" microflora on first six-week trials, in which case second-time trials may not be effective, as the "good-guys" microflora is not present in sufficient numbers to metabolize the medicine properly.

Supplementation with viable *Lactibacilus acidophilus* will normalize gut flora and reduce the concentration of gram-negative bacteria, a major source of "endotoxins." Endotoxins are toxins usually confined inside the body of a gram-negative bacterium until it dies, at which time it is released. At the same time Lactibacilus will inhibit overgrowth of *Candida albicans* which has itself been implicated in disruption of immune functions as well as GI inflammation, which could then increase absorption of existing endotoxins.

Such is not true of Clotrimazole and Tinidazole as these similar chemicals can be metabolized by both the human enzyme system and intestinal microflora. It's probably still best to supplement your diet with *Lactibacilus acidophilus* for many reasons, which we cover in other publications.

As a matter of good practice, after the initial few weeks of build-up of 5 to 6 one-quarter teaspoons per day, it might be well to supplement with the same 1/4 teaspoon about three to four times a day until you are certain that you no longer need the organism or other microflora that your physician suggests. In any case, it is well to take a dosage with every application of Metronidazole. Your physician may have different dosages in mind, which you should follow.

Incidentally, there is no evidence that Metronidazole when used intravenously has any effect on halting RD, but it does very quickly, and for a period, knock out inflammation that shows itself as swelling and heat. Metronidazole is used intravenously frequently for bacterial infections, especially when the patient has been hospitalized.

Do not take any kind of alcohol when taking these medicines. Metronidazole with even a small amount of alcohol, for example, acts as an anabuse, i.e., a substance used to make one sick enough to quit drinking alcohol. Alan Gaby, M.D. has also pointed out that some vinegars contain a small amount of alcohol, and so taking a salad with these vinegars as a dressing, along with Metronidzole, will make one quite sick.

The Physician's Desk Reference is often mis-interpreted as providing a single standard for administration of drugs, in the belief that only those diseases described therein can be treated by the associated drugs. I want to clarify that this book is simply a collection of drug package inserts placed there by pharmaceutical companies for the benefit of physician, pharmacist and patient in knowing what is being purchased and consumed. These package inserts, with their statements discussing characteristics and possible dangers of taking various medicines, are required by the U.S. Food and Drug Administration. In addition to scientific findings reported therein, any **possible** danger, whether known to be frequent or not, is contained therein. To gain FDA approval for release of a particular drug, for the medicinal use the company is promoting, the pharmaceutical company will include many symptoms that seem to occur when taking the drug, including some very rare effects and some symptoms virtually speculative. Whether or not a medicine is traditionally used by physicians for other purposes is seldom mentioned. In particular, if a medicine is being touted by the drug company as, say, an anti-bacterial agent, they have no responsibility to report that it is also used for an anti-protozoal, viral-static, or anti-viral agent.

68

The *Physician's Desk Reference,* in it's "Foreword to the Fortieth First Edition" (1987) states, "The FDA has also announced that the FD & C Act (Federal Drug and Cosmetic Act) 'does not, however, limit the manner in which a physician may use an approved drug. Once a product has been approved for marketing, a physician may prescribe it for uses or in treatment regimens or patient populations that are not included in approved labeling.'

Thus, the FDA states also that 'accepted medical practice' often includes drug use that is not reflected in approved drug testing."

So, when someone tells you that, say, Metronidazole is an antibacterial agent, or that Clotrimazole is mainly an "anti-fungal" agent, and that "everyone knows" that

Rheumatoid Arthritis is not caused by bacteria or fungus, just nod and go on your way. Many of the medicines listed above can be shown under laboratory conditions to be combinations of anti-bacterial, anti-viral, viral-static or anti-protozoal or antiyeast/fungus, under the correct conditions.

In the United States, the most frequently used first-trial medicine for Rheumatoid Disease (RD) is Metronidazole. It is listed in the *Physician's Desk Reference* as being FDA approved for marketing and human use. It is easily available by prescription and is relatively well known. It's use has resulted in a large number of remissions/cures.

To some extent Clotrimazole is anti-amoebic, anti-viral, viralstatic, anti-yeast/fungus, and anti-bacterial. It does not kill all germs, but for certain species, Clotrimazole may be effective in specific dosages under specific conditions.

Clotrimazole also inhibits a substance inside the body known as phospholipase A[2] which is a precursor (forerunner) to production of prostaglandins (from the arachidonic acid cascade) that helps to create inflammatory responses that produce heat (pyrexia), swelling (edema) and pain. Phospholipase is an enzyme derived from a fatty acid containing phosphorus.

Clotrimazole stimulates the body's own production of cortisol. It acts as an "immuno-modulator" changing some of the out-of-kilter characteristics o f the immunological system.

It kills *Candida albicans*, the yeast-fungus organism that causes so many symptoms that appear to be Rheumatoid Arthritis, and which also creates other major medical problems which is explained later.

Clotrimazole is usually easier for the patient to tolerate than Metronidazole — but patients vary.

So, which is the "best" medicine in the whole treatment protocol so far as is known to date?

Answer: There is no "best." The medicine that gets you well is best, and that may also vary from person to person.

For now be satisfied that a good honest trial of one (and possibly all) of the given medicines is your "best" opportunity to defeat the crippler than anything else available.

The Herxheimer Effect

Many traditional medical treatments require a trial and error period, just like ours. the physician evaluates effectiveness of a treatment by observing signs and clinical symptoms, and health progress. With our treatment, both the patient and the physician will know, after starting it, whether or not the treatment will <u>probably</u> be effective.

Usually, when one of the medicines is administered for RD, there will be a set of clinical signs and symptoms called the Jarisch-Herxheimer effect. Observing the Jarisch-Herxheimer effect, hereafter known as "The Herxheimer" is often very important for following the effectiveness of our treatment.

In 1902 two research physicians, Doctors Adolph Jarisch and Karl Herxheimer, studied the treatment of syphilis, using various kinds of relatively dangerous medicines. They learned that whenever they killed the syphilis spirochete the patient displayed a series of symptoms similar to "flu." They later concluded that whenever an organism more complex than a simple bacteria was killed within the human body, one had these same symptoms. Subsequently this phenomenon became named the "Jarisch-Herxheimer" or "Herxheimer" effect.

When treating tuberculosis, the Herxheimer occurs, as it also does in treating Leishmaniasis — some Desert Storm infections. When treating Leprosy, the same phenomenon occurs, but it is called "Lucio's" phenomenon." Some other rare, tropical diseases also exhibit the Herxheimer when treated by killing the causative organism. When treating *Candida albicans* it is called the "die off effect."

According to the Jarisch-Herxheimer theory, when an invading organism (more complex than a simple bacteria) acts as an antigen (allergy agent) the body prepares antibodies that tend to fight the antigen. This creates products which are the cause of the swelling, heat, and joint damage. One responds to the killing of the organism inside the body by having a serious allergic response inside the body. The products of that allergic response create secondary problems that lead to the additional damage.

If there is a causative organism that creates RD, and if the organism is killed by our medicine, and if a human has been sensitized to the protein products of that organism, then more of the protein products resulting from dead organisms will increase the internal allergic response. It follows, therefore, that the body will have an intensification of the very symptoms that we label as Rheumatoid Arthritis (RA).

Rheumatoid Arthritis symptoms are an external manifestation of the internal allergy!

Whenever a physician trained in our protocol treats a patient for Rheumatoid Disease, he/she looks very closely to observe if the patient is or is not having a Herxheimer. Usually, within a matter of a day or so the Herxheimer will occur if the treatment is to be successful. Such generality cannot be a golden rule, because there are a number of former arthritics who have had to take the medicine as long as six or seven weeks prior to observing a Herxheimer, and some few have Herxheimers that do not seem to terminate.

There are some, like I was, who are so sick at the time of treatment that neither the doctor nor patient are able to discriminate between the on-going disease and the Herxheimer. That is rare, however, and the normal case that is to respond will show the Herxheimer within a matter of days of treatment. A very few patients will get better without experiencing anything but a very light Herxheimer

— which they might not notice — but this is not the norm.

As reported by Gus J. Prosch, M.D. (deceased) of Birmingham, AL, the Herxheimer signs and symptoms are:

a. General and usual: Sweating and especially night sweats, diarrhea, nausea, vomiting, headache, fever, general malaise, flushing of skin, anorexia, aching bones and "flu" symptoms resembling a serum reaction.

b. The inflamed and affected tissues become more inflamed and tissues previously unknown to be involved become inflamed.

c. If the heart, pericardium or cardiac tissues are infected, patients may develop some paroxysmal auricular tachycardia, premature ventricular contractions or ectopic beats.

d. If the urinary bladder tissues are infected the patient may develop signs of full-blown cystitis.

e. If the brain or meninges are infected the patient may develop severe (temporary) depression, lethargy, generalized weakness, temporary memory loss, irritability along with headaches.

f. If the mouth tissues are infected, a bitter and/or metallic taste may be noted along with mild shedding or peeling of the mucosal tissues. This has also been noted in the rectal tissues. However, it should be noted that Metronidazole and Tinidazole also produce a metallic taste without the Herxheimer effect being present.

g. When the periosteal tissues and skeletal muscle tissues are involved, fairly severe bone pain usually accompanied by severe muscle pains and spasms may be observed, usually at night.

h. When the lungs and bronchial tissues are infected the patients may develop bronchitis symptoms and occasionally pneumonitis (resembling viral) has been observed.

From the above, Dr. Prosch stated, one can easily see that most all of the previously observed side effects of the recommended medicines may also be simply manifestations of the Herxheimer reaction. Therefore a clinician that is not totally knowledgeable concerning these possible signs and symptoms could easily mistake the Herxheimer reaction for possible side effects of the medicine. Should this information not be taken into consideration, a misleading and false evaluation of any adverse experiences by various patients caused by the medicine will be inevitable. The medicine could be labeled more dangerous than it actually may be, and the aggravated symptoms could get misconstrued as an intensification of the disease being treated. The information and the above facts **must be considered** in evaluating the medicine's effectiveness and side effects, when treating patients.

While the medicines may have a toxicity of their own — and in large dosages they surely do have — the symptoms listed in the *Physician's Desk Reference* are probably in many instances a report on the Herxheimer reaction rather than actual drug toxicity. The proof is that when a patient takes the medicine, and passes through the Herxheimer, the same drug dosage no longer produces the symptoms described on the package insert.

Professor Roger Wyburn-Mason's hypothesis that there exists a causative organism for Rheumatoid Disease which is more complex than a simple bacteria bears fruit. Once the Herxheimer is achieved, and the body cleans out the dead protein products (if that is what they are) and toxins, the individual gets well; i.e., the symptoms of swelling (edema), heat (pyrexia), night sweats, and increasing number of joint pains disappear, along with lethargy and depression.

From personal experience, and even though I knew full well better, during a course of a particular medicine, I have condemned and blamed the medicine as being the "cause" of my agony, the Herxheimer.

Afterwards, on cleaning out the debris within my body, I have felt wonderful, and the medicine in the same dosage is now seen as obviously not the cause of the Herxheimer. "Cleaning out the debris" means giving the body an opportunity to metabolize and/or eliminate toxins and other allergenic products.

Proof of Efficacy

A practicing physician could have treated 16,000 patients with great effectiveness, as did Jack Blount, Jr., M.D. Treating and achieving wellness for sixteen thousand, 20,000, . . . 100,000 patients are meaningless to the scientific medical community, unless those studies have been cast in the framework of double-blind studies, and subsequently accepted for publication in an accepted "peer-group," "refereed" medical journal. "Refereed" means that "peer" scientific physicians have an opportunity to search for scientific flaws in the article prior to being accepted for publication. Even then the publisher of a particular medical journal may, for reasons of bias or space or unknown reasons, reject the article for publication.

You can understand, then, that there is a great deal of political jockeying for space in such "peer group" journals, as publication therein can make reputations, and lead to better position and pay. There will be a tendency to build up respectability via the "buddy-buddy" system, as well as by "Authority," through "co-authoring" one another's articles. A big name on an article, along with the investigator 's, assures publication and often acceptance by the scientific community. The more a scientist gets published, the easier it is for the scientist to get published.

An ordinary practitioner of medicine has about as much chance of getting published in such "peer" group journals as the proverbial snowball surviving a day in hades, especially so when their chief dedication is toward helping patients, not in becoming an Authority.

What follows introduces patient treatment studies completed in a clinical setting by three different physicians in three different locations, with three different practices. Each physician making his own study wanted to satisfy himself that they were helping folks, and so, for their own purposes, they accumulated statistics in a setting that is not accepted as "proof" by authoritarian standards or "accepted" "peergroup" standards. But proof it nonetheless is, and a bright beacon in a sea of mysery!

Dr. Blount had had crippling Rheumatoid Disease since childhood. When he discovered Roger Wyburn-Mason's work, he was already bed-ridden, unable to walk, alcoholic, on drugs to kill the eternal pain and prepared to die. Trials of Metronidazole made him well. He called in a dozen elderly former patients giving them the opportunity to try the drug. Most of those who stayed with the treatment also got well. He reopened his practice and treated with great effectiveness another group of RD patients in excess of 16,000, including myself. As a former RD victim Dr. Blount was more familiar with the disease and its progress than most physicians, and it was quite obvious to him that the treatment was working on the vast majority of his patients.

William Renforth, M.D. of Connersville, IN published his studies in 1977. His successes are reported in our *Historical Documents in Search for the Cure for Rheumatoid Disease*[2].

Gus J. Prosch, Jr. had a successful medical trial on his back problem that traditional practices stated would require an operation. Dr. Blount had suggested he try Metronidazole and Allopurinol first, as Dr. Prosch could always have the operation if the medicine did not help. The treatment was successful in ridding Dr. Prosch of his back pain for the first time in 7 years. On behalf of his patients, Dr. Prosch felt an obligation to study his patient's case histories and to compile their statistics.

Robert Bingham, M.D. (deceased) on the other hand, had specialized as an orthopaedic surgeon and general practitioner with polio victims and later arthritic victims, the latter for more than 30 years. He therefore knew success and non-success quite well. Through his long years of experience he further had an ability to separate out various kinds of arthritic characteristics (signs and symptoms) and could, therefore, pre-select patients who would most likely respond to Rheumatoid Disease protocols.

Dr. Paul K. Pybus, (deceased) our former Chief Medical Advisor, worked under the supervision of Roger Wyburn-Mason, M.D. in his youth, and had learned to respect the physician's brilliance and originality in medicine. Pybus investigated Wyburn-Mason's claims, tried the treatments, and was convinced by his patient's results. Dr. Pybus often published his observations as

"Letters" in the *South African Medical Journal* or the English published *Lancet*.

Statistics compiled by Prosch, Bingham and Pybus follow:

PARTIAL REPORT OF SUMMARY OF TREATING PATIENTS WITH MEDICATION

Gus J. Prosch, Jr., M.D.

Effect	Metronidazole	%	Furoxone	%	Rimactane	%
None	7	3.5	23	39.0	16	5.0
Mild	9	4.5	7	11.9	5	16.0
Moderate	29	14.5	5	8.5	3	9.0
Good	56	28.0	14	23.7	5	16.0
Very Good	99	49.5	10	16.9	3	9.0
Total	**200**	**100**	**59**	**100**	**32**	**55**

COMPARATIVE RESULTS OF TREATMENT WITH OTHER DRUGS

Robert Bingham, M.D.

Treatment	Patients Treated	Improved or Remissions	Percent Change
Controls	22	7	31
Conventional Care	30	8	27
Copper Sulfate	12	8	66
Bile Salts	12	9	75
Clotrimazole	9	7	78
Diiodohydroxyquion	204	189	93
Chloroquine	12	6	50
Metronidazole	221	181	82*

Patients   Improved or Percent

*Recent cases [at the time of this report] have done better on increased dosages.

CLINICAL RESULTS IN 156 PATIENTS

Dr. Paul K. Pybus

Clinical Results	Number	Percent
Poor (no change)	11	7
Fair (slightly improved)	35	22
Good (one joint still troublesome)	60	38
Excellent (symptomless)	50	32

Nineteen years (1996) have passed since these studies were made. Subsequent follow-up data passed to me orally from those physicians who tally their clinical results indicated a <u>consistent</u> 80% success rate in patient healing, the one exception being the 50% subgroup success rate noted for those that have already been abused by gold, penicillamine, methotrexate (cytotoxic drugs) and long-term corticosteroids. Adding additional, safe, treatments, as described herein, can effectively "cure" virtually all rheumatoid victims.

Previously I reported on the "placebo" effect in the treating of arthritics, and that it was 30%. This means that any scientific statistical study must account for about 30% of the patients responding well — or at least appearing to

— for reasons to do with mood, natural variations between humans, "belief" or "faith" or reasons just unknown. No matter what a physician does the patient will show "improvement" at least temporarily.

Look closely at the statistics offered. Study them. There can be no explanation for the great differences between an anticipated placebo effect of 30% and the <u>consistent</u>

80% success rate, or better, displayed by different physicians in far different clinical settings with much different backgrounds and experiences! — other than to conclude the extremely high probability that this treatment protocol is 165%, or greater, better than traditional treatments, and safer than traditional Rheumatology practices which, remember, do not claim to cure or permanently improve anyone, but do claim to get about 30% "improvement," at least temporarily. Note that the 30% placebo effect is exactly the same figure as the

30% temporary "improvement" effect achieved in traditional practices. (For the source of the 30% figure, read *Clinics in Rheumatic Diseases*, December 1983, published by W.B. Saunders, a peer-group accepted publication informing practicing rheumatologists of the state-of-art of their treatment protocols as scientifically evaluated.)

There are some patients, it should be mentioned in passing, who will get well permanently no matter what is done. Medical science does not explain this, other than to label it as a "spontaneous remission" which is a scientific name substituted for the term "faith cure" used by various religious groups.

We are quite happy for wellness in former victims, no matter how labeled or to whom they attribute their great relief.

Additional Treatment Requirements

It is <u>essential</u> that other components of our treatment protocol also be followed, and these include nutritional aspects, treatment for Candidiasis, food allergy treatments, possible Chelation Therapy, and many other possible health improving treatments.

See our summary at the end of this book.

References

1. *Physician's Desk Reference,* Medical Economics Company, Inc., Oradell, N.J. 07649, 1987.

2. *Historical Documents in Search for the Cure for*

Rheumatoid Disease, www.arthritistrust.org, 1985.

Proper Nutrition for Rheumatoid Arthritis

When using the Rheumatoid Disease Foundation's treatment protocol, or anyone else's treatment protocol, proper nutrition is essential for arthritics. In fact, the foundation to proper healing for any disease condition is that of proper nutrition.

Rheumatoid Arthritis (collagen tissue disease) victims, however, may require special attention to certain nutrients, such as the proper Essential Fatty Acids, and also possible additional vitamin and mineral supplements, including the various anti-oxidants, and perhaps even boron, an element once thought not to have any use by the human body, but determined by the research of Rex E. Newnham, Ph.D., D.O., N.D. (deceased) to be vital for all arthritics and reported in our article, *Boron and Arthritis*[13].

Gus J. Prosch, Jr., M.D. has long advised patients on proper nutritional supplements and diets. In his *Essential Fatty Acids are Essential*[14], we have printed the relationship between certain foods and the influence on our bodies of oils derived from those foods. His information is also extremely important for arthritics.

There have been many books written over several generations on the subject of nutrition as it relates to Rheumatoid Arthritis — and probably many of them are correct, for some people.

Some physicians and health oriented advisors will take the stand that nutrition alone can cure arthritis, and they also may be correct under certain conditions. It obviously happens with sufficient frequency for the truth to linger, but not with high enough frequency to convince all of us who have tragically become victims of the crippler.

What I believe happens is this: Major factors that contribute to the precipitation of Rheumatoid Disease (RD) are genetic, stress, and weakening of the immunological system. Many people are under continuing stress, thus weakening their ability to fight off infection and Rheumatoid Arthritis. Several kinds of stress exist, including emotional, physical and nutritional.

Whenever we RD-prone folks ignore good nutritional habits over long periods, our bodies lose ability to produce the necessary fighting tools to ward off physical and emotional problems and also we lose the ability to repair tissues and organs properly under normal wear and tear. We generate "free radicals," chemicals that have the need for more electrons and which easily, quickly attach to other cellular molecules that would be better off without the additional burdens. These free radicals disturb our bodily functions, and inhibit our ability to repair ourselves, or to restore our good health.

If Rheumatoid Disease begins at this point, and if the individual returns to a good and proper diet at once, and if the individual knowingly or unknowingly reduces the critical stress, then I believe the regression of Rheumatoid Arthritis is much more likely without any further treatment — but not certain!

What is probably normal is that stress continues onward — we are unable to leave a particularly detested job, weighty family responsibilities seem unsolvable, children continue to perplex us with their persistent problems, the husband or wife is a "suppressive personality," constantly undercutting our beingness, and so on.

Under such circumstances perhaps no amount of good nutritional habits will help the genetically predisposed arthritic.

More than likely, the arthritic continues on with the same poor food habits of a lifetime, and so nutritional aspects are ignored in any case.

Perhaps either relief of stress or improved nutrition, or combinations of both stress relief and improved nutrition "spontaneously" brings about remission of the disease. About 1/3 of those first afflicted seem to recover "spontaneously," at least for the time being.

Usually the initial plea for help is to the rheumatologist who, being trained in the traditional and "time-honored" "accepted" treatments (treating symptoms, not causes), first provides costly tests, presumably confirming the condition of arthritis. Then secondly aspirin is tried. When aspirin no longer helps (or becomes dangerous in quantities needed to suppress pain symptoms) he/she writes prescriptions for NSAIDS (non-steroidal anti-inflammatories). When these fail to control pain — and they eventually will — he/she advises use of dangerous gold shots which not only have damaging side-effects but in any case will not be effective — if at all — beyond thirty months. When this fails or proves too toxic for a patient to tolerate, penicillamine is used, and after that methotrexate. All of this will or will not accompany the increasing use of cortico-steroids in ever heavier dosages

— and sickness rages onward!

Having failed in this direction, from light to heavy symptomatic treatments, peer-group practicing rheumatologists have now begun to lean in the other direction, begining first with the most dangerous, and the most damaging cytotoxic drugs. They arrived at this decision via vote, such is the measure of their "scientific medicine."

There are two accepted possible hypothesis for the causation of Rheumatoid Arthritis (as opposed to the possibility of a multiplicity of causes). These are that (1) something is wrong with the immunological system; and (2) that some organism, unknown, creates an internal "allergic" response which manifests itself as the symptoms of Rheumatoid Arthritis. While the second guess may be wrong, at least there is often success in following treatments that derive from that clue; whereas there is never success in the first guess. Why a defect in someone's immunological system should suggest that we deliberately damage his/her immunological system further, as happens with cytotoxic drugs, gold, penicillamine and longterm cortico-steroids has never been satisfactorily explained by rheumtologists.

The peer group publication, *Clinics in Rheumatic Diseases*[1] is a scientific standard for evaluating clinical applications. It clearly shows that gold shots when subjected to standards of double-blind tests failed the pre-defined criteria by 1% but was accepted as a symptomatic "safe and effective" treatment nonetheless. After thirty months, the symptomatic "effectiveness" fails almost completely. The studies, of course, do not dwell on the tremendous toxicity when using the drug, nor on the fact that after its use, the immunological system may be damaged.

The same publication presents the fact that there is absolutely no scientific evidence for the use of penicillamine, yet that is the substance often prescribed after gold fails. Penicillamine, of course, is also toxic and dangerous.

One doctor believes that the chief advantage to use of penicillamine after use of gold is the fact that it is a chelator (removes out) for the gold. A build up of gold in the bodily tissues contributes to increasing toxicities which add to the arthritic symptoms and burdens. The two symptoms — toxicity of gold and RD symptoms — appear to the patient (and doctor) as symptoms of progressive Rheumatoid Disease. When gold is no longer even marginally helpful, the physician, knowledgeably or otherwise, in resorting to penicillamine chelates out (removes out) some of the toxic gold, thus giving the patient a sense of improvement as the symptoms due to toxicity of the gold is lifted from his/her tissues.

Of course, the Rheumatoid Disease rages onward. When penicillamine fails, Methotrexate, or some other dangerous cytotoxic drug is often next, and it is a most dangerous and futile drug. I would challenge any physician to demonstrate that this drug, or any of those listed above will cure or bring about long-range remission of arthritis in any number of significant cases in quantities greater than the normal placebo effect of 30%!

It is most probable that had the rheumatologist instead concentrated on helping the patient to learn about and relieve stress and also to change dietary habits, the percentage of successes would have been greater than the placebo effect of 30%. This approach would have taken a great deal of extra time, at greater sacrifice of the physician's income. Sadly for our society, most physicians are taught by medical schools to treat symptoms, not causes, which results in the administering of drugs to relieve symptoms, not in searching out causes and teaching the patient to understand the stresses of his/her immediate environment. While this approach serves well pharmaceutical companies, and keeps patients returning to the physician's office, it cannot cure.

This accepted rheumatology treatment process is rather hard on you and me.

Meanwhile it is difficult, if not impossible, to purchase the food that our bodies require from restaurants and quick-food franchises. While dieticians and corporate stock advisors explain how nutritious the local hamburger joint is, you and I as arthritics should be better educated and behave accordingly.

Nutrition for Arthritics

Like most folks I like mother's cooking best. She's deceased and I still like her recipes best. What you and I like to eat is what we've been conditioned to like from childhood, not of choice. Because we are able to make a choice, and because we always choose what we like best — mother's cooking — does not mean that we have exercised that free choice, but rather that we have determined our choices by our likes which were determined by our earlier conditioning — before we had a choice — which is no longer "free choice."

Since becoming a victim of arthritis I've read many books on nutrition, but I will not pretend to be a nutrition expert. Possibly one reason that the subject of proper nutrition is not taught in medical schools -- or underemphasized if it is taught — is that it is the most complex of medical subjects, requiring far more knowledge of the human biochemistry than modern day undergraduate medical schools can provide.

There are hundreds of good books[3] on nutrition, but not all books on good nutrition are really about good nutrition. The old fashioned method of stating that all you need for good health is the four basic food groups, or the six groups or whatever the latest buzzwords happen to be is misleading. No successful farmer would feed his cows, chickens or hogs without careful consideration to total nutrient needs. To do otherwise would invite bankruptcy. The human body, being composed of similar physiological functions and elements, needs no less consideration.

In Maureen Salaman's *The Cancer Answer*[2] excellent points are made that the closer we can get to eating as did our primitive forefathers, the healthier we shall be. After all, our bodies are the product of millions of years of evolution in conjunction with other organisms such as plants and animals. We have, through this joint-evolution, adapted, just as plants and other animals have adapted to our precursors.

A rather excellent book by Sally Fallon, Pat Connolly and Mary G. Enig, Ph.D., *Nourishing Traditions*,[17]

provides understandable reasons for eating properly, as well as many excellent recipes for preparing our food properly.

"Normal" Diets vary worldwide and encompass for humans almost everything edible and safe, whether insect, mammal, cacti, fungi, eel, snake, fish, tuber. . . .

In addition to our very early conditioning and the daily barrage of huxterism by food processing monopolies and fast food franchises, there is the fact that more and more polluting chemicals are being spread on our crops even as trace elements in our soils disappear. How food is shipped, stored and handled or processed affects nutrition values. The food that looks so healthy on supermarket shelves may not be so nutritious on laboratory analysis. So we, as arthritics, are faced with another problem: Where to get food that is wellness-forming?

Speaking of modern-day food sources, one article by specialists in biochemistry and nutrition starts out like this: There are two kinds of things that people place in their mouths and eat. One of these we shall call "food," and the other we shall call "non-food," We shall define "non-food" as every kind that is packaged, processed, refined, or otherwise changed from its natural form. This will include all canned goods, all dried fruits and vegetables, frozen foods, all sterilized and otherwise cooked foods that are then cooled and sold in supermarkets, all irradiated foods, and so on. Candies, gums, cakes, pies and such mixtures are also "non-food." Quite obviously plastic and chemical substitutes for foods are not foods. Examples of these are margarine (more a plastic than anything else, and even insects have a sufficient instinct to ignore it); imitation ice-cream, fake eggs, imitation whipped cream and so on.

So what is left to be called "food"?

Well, fresh fruits and vegetables, nuts, whole grains, fresh poultry, beef, lamb and pork and so on.

Incidentally, by this definition of "food," vitamins are not foods, as they are the result of having been processed or synthesized, but this category is an exception to the general rule stated, to ignore "non-foods." As the soils have been depleted of essential minerals, that everything during the preparation, packaging, transportation, and sale of the product is aimed at extending the shelf-life of perishable products, to the vast detriment of the nutritional content of the product, vitamins and minerals are increasingly necessary for maintenance of good health, and especially so the various antioxidants.

The point is that "food" is nature's complete package container that has not only a lot of nutritional elements that we need and know about, but also a lot of food elements that we need and don't know about, particularly trace minerals, enzymes and compounds that our body will utilize for processes unknown. Processing nature's package for the purpose of preserving shelf-life destroys necessary compounds and enzymes or eliminates trace elements.

Each of us was created uniquely and endowed genetically differently, which means that each of us has different nutritional requirements in addition to a commonalty of nutritional requirements. Anyone who is dogmatic about what you need, and tells you that you need only so and so in certain amounts to be healthy is probably mistaken, just as the standard minimum daily requirements of vitamins and minerals when applied to the individual are usually mistaken.

The reason that the minimum daily requirements (or Recommended Daily Allowance, RDA) as to daily amount required is usually wrong is because such figures represent averages of groups of people, not a unique individual requirement for you. Some folks require far, far more Vitamin D than others, and can tolerate enough that would poison others, some may require less. Whenever a physician or know-it-all academician tells you that you <u>must</u> or <u>must not</u> take a certain amount of a vitamin or mineral each day to be healthy, in the absence of specific information about you, he/she is ignorant of individual differences and how the minimum daily requirements (or RDA) were ascertained.

For the most part, the standards of minimum daily requirements for vitamins and minerals were established as <u>lower</u> boundaries to prevent disease states, like scurvy,

not to define quantities required to furnish individualized wellness!

Neither can anyone guess at what foods you should eat, and how much, except in special circumstances where disease states are to be prevented, and certain requirements are well known outside of your individualized biochemistry.

Consider vitamin C, for example. As you are probably aware, there has been much controversy over the usage of vitamin C in larger or smaller quantities. Only certain mammals besides man are incapable of producing their own vitamin C. Did you ever wonder how so many animals, like dogs and cats, can eat garbage and disease-ridden foods and remain healthy? It is because God has found in his wisdom that their bodies shall produce the chemicals required to fight off infection and poisons, and vitamin C is a requisite part of that system.

As described in our *Vitamin C: How to Use The Great Missing Vitamin*[3], Robert F. Cathcart, M.D. has shown that each individual, at different times during the day, and on differing days, require differing amounts of vitamin C to handle stress, disease and other physiological problems.

It becomes clearer with the study of various dietary recommendations, that Maureen Salaman's "cave-man diet" (*The Cancer Answer*[2]) recommendations and Sally Fallon's "cook book" (*Nourishing Traditions*[17]) should be read by all lay people.

Another very excellent book, written by Sherry A. Rogers, M.D., is *Wellness Against All Odds*[10]. Dr. Rogers, after many years of experience with many dietary programs, remarkably concludes that different diets fit different people, at different times.

As people grow, mature, and become old, they require differing quantities of different foods. Different disease states require differing quantities. The field of nutrition and nutritional supplements is indeed complex — too complex for simplistic answers given by health professionals who have had virtually no — or very little — training on the subject in medical schools.

What is wrong with our diets is easier to answer: According to William Campbell Douglass, M.D., we Americans consume 18 percent of our calories as refined sugar which has no vitamins or minerals necessary for metabolism. We consume another 18 percent of our calories in the form of refined, enriched white flour which is nutritionally deficient in about 28 essential nutrients, including vitamin B[3]. Nancy Appleton, Ph.D. in her *Lick The Sugar Habit*, devastates the industry with facts and figures on the damage done by sugar in the American diet[4]. The Price-Pottenger Nutrition Foundation[5] is an excellent source for nutritional information (*Nourishing Traditions*[17]).

Although there are some well-known general principles to use as guides for good health through nutrition, there are no easy answers. You must solve the nutritional riddle yourself, hopefully with the help of a knowledgeable health professional. If you can't grow proper food, you must find the best fresh fruit and vegetables possible, and you should probably supplement your diet in ways that are guided by the best nutritionally oriented physician possible. Additionally you should read books about the nutritional aspects of arthritis. The Price-Pottenger Nutrition Foundation[5] is also an excellent source for this purpose.

Having stated some of the general principles that apply, and my personal conclusions, I now go on to our treatment protocol respecting nutrition.

The Arthritis Trust of America's/The Rheumatoid Disease Foundation's Nutritional Recommendations

Having first had this Foundation's treatment for Rheumatoid Disease, and having halted disease progress, I was able to maintain my wellness state for but two to three months. Our treatment says to take a trial dosage of anti-amoebic (anti-microbial) drugs every six months to learn if one again has the Herxheimer, indicating renewal of the disease. If so, one is to then take the full six week treatment. I found that I was taking the medicine every two to six months, and from time to time suffering for an evening or so with a severe Herxheimer reaction. (See our *The Herxheimer Effect*[7].)

Note that the Herxheimer reaction lasted, during these trial periods but an evening or so during which I was terribly sick to the point where I cared less if the world turned or not. But the next morning I would feel absolutely great again, and ready to tackle the lions of this world. As a precautionary measure, of course, I would complete the full treatment for six weeks.

I also received letters and talked to people having the same repeat cycle. We learned from a research pharmacologist that metabolization of metronidazole did not occur with natural stomach processes but rather required good intestinal microflora, and I therefore supplemented with *Lactibacilus acidophilus*, but that obviously was not the complete answer. (We also learned from Alan Gaby, M.D., that some vinegars used on salads containe small amounts of alcohol, and alcohol combined with metronidazole, one of our recommended medicines, acted as an anabuse, i.e., a terrible reaction which drives people away from the use of alcohol. Thus, vinegars were to be avoided while taking metronidazole.)

To be "cured" meant to me not to have a return of the disease.

Physicians will accept a "cure" of tonsillitis, and call its return as "another infection" -which was not good enough for me with a disease that might still lead to crippling each time it returned.

We arthritics will not be satisfied with two to three months halt in disease progress, although that is infinitely better than no halt at all.

And so, during those early Rheumatoid Disease Foundation days we continued our search for a better answer for ourselves, in addition to pushing to the limit of our resources various university medical research.

Some of our referral physicians constantly spoke to us about the importance of diet, which we ignored, as some of our other physicians who are not diet oriented still do.

I, like you, was severely conditioned by mother's cooking. I also believed the authoritarian attitude of physicians who were generally unlearned respecting nutrition, but rather prescribed pills and shots for everything — the symptomatic approach — treat symptoms and ignore the cause! Usually their uninformed doggerel supports the idea that "your present diet, consisting of the four food groups, furnishes you with all necessary vitamins and minerals."

False!

At last I paid attention to the diet requirements for arthritics. The principles are quite simple to state.

The intestinal track must have acidity (hydrochloric acid) to properly utilize food and prevent overgrowth of "bad-guys" microflora. Other bodily tissues should be slightly alkaline, rather than acidic. A simple test developed by Carl Reich, M.D. (deceased)[11] of Canada using pH litmus paper told me that my saliva was exceedingly acidic, whereas testing of other healthy people, children and friends, found that their saliva was slightly alkaline.

A test that you can easily perform is this: Purchase a small amount of litmus paper through your pharmacy. When a child has not eaten for an hour or so — no liquids or food -- place their saliva on it. Do the same with a healthy teen-ager, and then another healthy adult, and also yourself. You will most probably find the youngest has a very dark purple, and then the color decreases with age, shades of purple become lighter until you reach yourself, where yours will be of no color at all. The test which is easy to repeat on many others as well as yourself will demonstrate that as we grow older and more careless of our diet, our saliva becomes more acidic. This test is also a very good monitoring device over many months of diet change, to determine if you are indeed making progress with the right kinds of healthier foods.

It took me two years — mostly of procrastinating (remember my mother's early conditioning) — before I turned this test about, and also sustained permanency in relief from the arthritic condition!

To eat properly at last, I followed the Gus Prosch, Jr., M.D. advice. Dr. Prosch was also a specialist in clinical nutrition.

Although I haven't always adhered strictly to a good diet since, I haven't had a recurrence of Rheumatoid Arthritis in more than nineteen years.

As all Rheumatoid Arthritis victims also suffer from Candidiasis (*Candida albicans*) Dr. Prosch says that the Candidiasis diet, being more restrictive than a general arthritic diet, should probably be followed first. Food allergies will follow from Candidiasis, and so one must also enter into elimination diets and biodetoxification regimens[15].

Dr. Gus J. Prosch's Dietary Recommendations for the Rheumatoid Arthritic[12]

Dr. Prosch tells his patients, the following: "I would like to discuss the importance of diet, nutrition and vitamin and mineral supplementation in Rheumatoid Disease patients. Many different opinions and conclusions among most physicians today are fairly rampant and many doctors do not believe this subject is important, so I'm going to tell you about my beliefs and observations as to how and why I treat my patients.

"In my observations and research there are several things that to me stand out to be quite significant in most patients with Rheumatoid Disease.

"1. The great majority of Rheumatoid Disease patient's body fluids are too acid in nature.

"2. The great majority of these patients show signs and symptoms of a deficiency in free or ionic calcium.

"3. Most Rheumatoid Disease patients eat margarine instead of butter

"3. and they demonstrate a lack of Vitamin A and natural D deficiencies of the essential fatty acids. plus severe

"4. Diet in Rheumatoid Disease does help control the severity of the symptoms.

"5. Vitamin and mineral supplementations help shorten the recovery time by strengthening the immune system.

"In studying the nutrition status and diet of Rheumatoid Disease patients, I made three observations that have caused me to look deeper into this subject.

"1. I observed that many patients who are blood-related to arthritic patients do not develop any arthritis especially when different dietary habits were followed.

"2. I observed that often-times arthritic patients exhibited slight to significant improvement when self-administered home and folk remedies were taken, like alfalfa tablets, bone meal tablets, cod liver oil, vinegar with honey, peanut oil, . . . or cherries.

"3. I observed that some arthritic patients are more susceptible to getting reinfected after being treated with the medication that apparently eliminated the offending organisms.

"I found by checking the acidity of saliva and urine of arthritic patients, that the great majority were considerably more acid than normal and I concluded that an alkaline diet could only benefit these patients.

"I also found by careful observation that Rheumatoid Disease patients more often than normal exhibited certain physical signs during the physical examination. To summarize these signs, they are as follows:

"1. Longitudinal ridges and increased opaqueness in fingernails.

"2. Mild to moderate tenderness with strong palpation of the soleus or trapezius muscles.

"3. Generalized slight increase in deep tendon reflexes.

"4. Generalized irritability of skeletal muscles to percussion.

"5. Acid saliva of pH 4.5 to 6.5.

"6. Slight to severe coating on the tongue.

"Many of these signs are related to calcium metabolism in the body and most arthritic patients drink 2% or low fat milk and eat margarine instead of butter.

The previously mentioned physical signs demonstrate strong evidence of free or ionic calcium deficiency as well as a deficiency of Vitamin A and D which is natural Vitamin D. Blood calcium studies are misleading as they measure the ionic calcium as well as calcium bound to proteins. Whereas normal body fluids ideally are slightly alkaline as opposed to acid, and I believe the one primary cause of the deficiency in Rheumatoid Disease patients of the ionic calcium which in itself is very alkaline.

An even more important cause of this acidity is due to the diet and nutritional habits of these arthritic patients. Most cellular mechanisms of the body and particularly those involving the use of ionized minerals such as the secretory glands, nerve function processes and muscle contraction, etc. proceed best in a mildly alkaline state. For this reason a diet consisting of high alkaline foods should be consumed, combined with the avoidance of acid-forming foods.

"Acid-forming foods are those which are high in one or more of three elements: phosphorus, sulfur, and chlorine; alkaline diets are those high in potassium, calcium, magnesium and sodium.

"The diet used to treat and prevent development of Rheumatoid Diseases should definitely avoid as much as possible the following foods. All processed and most canned foods should be avoided along with caffeine, sugar in all it's forms, as well as the simple carbohydrate foods that quickly upon digestion turn into sugar, like white flour foods, crackers, many cereals, macaroni (pasta foods) white rice and corn products.

"Ideally nicotine and alcohol should be avoided, along with any sweets, candy, soft drinks, pastries and desserts.

"The 'nightshade plants' (foods containing solanines) such as white potatoes, tomatoes, egg plant and garden peppers should be avoided. (Robert Bingham, M.D. stated that about 1/3 of arthritics are sensitive to solanines.).

"As a rule, most protein foods tend to be acid forming since they contain phosphorus and sulfur. Animal sources of protein — lean meat (beef, lamb, veal) poultry, fish and eggs — are definitely in this category. With the exception of shrimp, most sea food is extremely acid forming. These foods must not be avoided in the diet, however, as they provide the building blocks for all bodily functions and processes. Therefore one of these proteins should be eaten with each meal. Pork meats should be limited however.

"Just try not to eat an entire meal consisting of protein foods, but balance these foods with alkaline forming foods. Ideally your breakfast should always consist of some high protein foods, balanced with whole milk, fruit juices, etc. Also remember to cook protein foods at low temperatures, as enzymes and trace minerals are reduced with excessive heat and no foods should be eaten that have been deep fried.

"Avoid processed and hydrogenated, or "hardened" oils and fats. Most margarines, peanut butters, restaurant prepared French fries and potato or corn chips are prepared with hardened oils.

"Sweet cream butter is best and use "cold pressed" vegetable oils or "Pam" for home cooking. Also watch those high calorie salad dressings. Most fats and fatty foods (butter, oils, sausages, bacon, etc.) are neutral in their acid-alkaline content but they greatly contribute to excessive weight gain which severely complicates arthritis. Therefore, it would be wise to limit all oily, greasy, fried, fatty foods if one tends to be overweight.

"Most all vegetables (except corn) are highly alkaline in nature and should be emphasized in the eating program. Salad vegetables are excellent and should be eaten daily. All other vegetables are very good and when "Wok" cooked or stir-fried in cold pressed vegetable oil are even better.

"Fresh vegetable juices (not canned) are nearly perfect and should be part of the diet. It is important to prepare and serve as many foods in their raw and natural state as possible.

"All fruits and fruit juices (excepting cranberries, plums and prunes) are alkaline forming and are good to 'munch' on.

"Whole milk is one of the best alkaline forming foods due to its high calcium content. Raw certified whole milk is much preferable if you can find it. (Unfortunately raw milk is available in very few states.) At least two glasses of whole milk should be taken each day.

"Plain yogurt is an excellent alkalinizing food and not only is easy to digest, but tastes great when mixed with fresh fruit such as raisins, dates, dried figs and apricots. It also makes excellent munching foods. (Watch out for packaged yogurt with fruit, as it often contains damaging sugar.)

"This diet will change one's system to be more alkaline as it should be.

"Concerning vitamin and mineral supplementation, the most important point to consider here is to correct the free calcium deficiency present in most arthritics. This requires much larger amounts of vitamin A and D in their natural form than what is usually recommended by the

'Recommended Daily Allowances' tables.

"The synthetic Vitamin A and D preparations on the market simply do not work. Synthetic Vitamin D does increase the calcium absorption from the small intestine but seems to be totally inadequate in regulating the use of the calcium and especially calcium excretion by the kidneys. The only preparation I have found that is adequate is the natural D which is found in fish liver oils. Therefore I recommend Norwegian Cod Liver Oil as the ideal which seems to be even better than cod liver oil capsules. It is easily taken when mixed with some orange juice and stirred rapidly. The preparation I recommend is plain Norwegian Cod Liver Oil liquid which contains 10,000 units of Vitamin A and 1000 units of Vitamin D per teaspoon. I recommend that patients take two teaspoons on arising each morning and two teaspoons at bedtime. This preparation can be found in most health food stores and should be taken for at least four months, then the dosage should be cut in half.

"I explain to the patients not to fear any Vitamin A or D toxicity with this dosage as it is less than 1/3 the toxicity level that has been reported in the literature. If the patient absolutely cannot take the liquid, they can usually find capsules at a health food store which will provide approximately 4,000 units of Vitamin D daily.

"I also explain that exposure to sunshine for at least 20 minutes each week will activate the Vitamin D. "Concerning the calcium preparations I have found that none of the available inorganic calcium preparations are effective. I discovered that organic bone meal tablets (3-4 per day) work better than other calcium preparations but I continued to have reservations. I located a calcium preparation which seems to work ideally. This compound is Calcium Orotate (500 mg 4 times daily). This calcium preparation also seems to enhance the ability of the body to use and metabolize other forms of calcium ingested. It is the naturally occurring Calcium in plants. Calcium Chelate or Calcium Aspartate can substitute, although most any Calcium is good except bone meal or Calcium Carbonate.

"I also have prescribed 500 mg of Magnesium Orotate twice daily to balance the calcium/magnesium ratio. The above calcium preparation is also excellent for osteoporosis and it greatly strengthens the bone and cartilage structures in the body.

"Concerning other vitamins for arthritic patients, I recommend as an ideal supplemental program the following:

"a. Vitamin B Complex, two to three 'Stress' B vitamins daily in divided doses. (These should contain 50-75 mg of each B vitamin).

"b. Vitamin C, two to three grams daily in divided doses.

"c. Zinc Orotate, 500 mg one to two tablets on an empty stomach or use Zinc Chelate or Zinc Aspartate.

"d. Selenium, 250 micrograms daily as yeast selenium.
"e. B-Carotene, 25,000 units daily.

"f. Vitamin E, 400 units daily.

The above vitamin and mineral supplementations will not only help the patient's arthritis by stimulating the immune response system but will play an important role in counteracting the aging process as well as acting as a deterrent to some forms of cancer since many of these preparations act as free radical and peroxide scavengers in the body.

"With painful hands and feet, I recommend in addition 100 mg Vitamin B . (Dosages may be much higher, 200 mg per day or more for 90 days, according to John Marion Ellis, M.D., who was able to prove, clinically and experimentally a B deficiency connection between loss of finger flexion, carpal tunnel syndrome and other physical problems[16].)"

References

1. *Clinics in Rheumatic Diseases*, W.B. Saunders & Co, December 1983, ISBN: 0307-742X.

2. Jeffrey Bland, Ph.D., *Medical Applications of Clinical Nutrition* edited by and published by Keats Publishing Co. ISBN: 087983-327-0 recommended for physicians; Maureen Salaman, President of the National Health Federation, has studied the issue of nutrition in Cancer. Her book, *The Cancer Answer* (ISBN: 0-913087-00-9) is a remarkable summary of the chief tenets of good nutrition, not just for arthritics, but for everyone. Stratford Publishing, 1259 El Camino Real, Suite 1500, Menlo Park, CA 94025.

3. William Campbell Douglass, M.D., *The Cutting Edge*, The Douglass Center, 2470 Windy Hill Road, Suite 440, Marietta, Ga 30067.

4. Nancy Appleton, Ph.D., *Lick the Sugar Habit*, Warner Books, Inc., 666 Fifth Avenue, New York, NY 10103, p. 1986.

5. Price/Pottenger Foundation, 5871 El Cajon Blvd, San Diego, CA 92115.

6. Robert F. Cathcart, M.D./Anthony di Fabio, *Vitamin C: The Great Missing Vitamin*, www.arthritistrust.org; *The Art of Getting Well*, www.arthritistrust.orgOp.Cit, 1985.

7. Dr. Paul K. Pybus/Anthony di Fabio, *The Herxheimer Effect*, www.arthritistrust.org, Op.Cit., 1992; *The Art of Getting* Well,www.arthritistrust.org Op.Cit., 1985,

8. Anthony di Fabio, *Candidiasis: The Scourge of Arthritics*, www.arthritistrust.orgOp.Cit., 1994; *The Art of Getting* Well, Kindle or Nook, Op.Cit., 1985;

9. Raul Vergini,M.D., *MagnesiumChloride HexahydrateTherapy*, www.arthritistrust.org, Op. Cit., 1994; *Townsend Letter for Doctors*, "Magnesium Chloride in acute & Chronic Diseases" (letter) #112, 1992, p. 992.

10. Sherry A. Rogers, M.D., *Wellness Against All Odds*, Prestige Publishing, Box 3068, 3500 Brewerton Rd., Syracuse, NY 13220, 1994.

11. Carl H. Reich, M.D. and Robert R. Barefoot, *The Calcium Factor: The Scientific Secret of Health and Youth*, Bokar Consultants (US) Inc., P.O. Box 21270, Wickenburg, AZ 85358, 1992.

12. Gus J. Prosch, Jr., M.D., "Dietary Recommendations for the Rheumatoid Arthritic." Transcribed with permission from The Rheumatoid Disease Foundation's Second Annual Medical

Convention, 1986; *Proper Nutrition for Rheumatoid Arthritis,* www.arthritistrust.org, Op.Cit., 1994.

13. Rex E. Newnham, Ph.D., D.O., N.D., Boron and Arthritis, www.arthritistrust.org, Op.Cit., 1994.

14. Gus J. Prosch, Jr., M.D., *Essential Fatty Acids are Essential,* www.arthritistrust.org, Op.Cit., 1994.

15. Warren Levin, M.D., Anthony di Fabio, *Allergies and Biodetoxification for the Arthritic,* www.arthritistrust.org, Op.Cit., 1994.

16. John Marion Ellis, M.D., *Free of Pain,* National headquarters Natural Food Associates, PO Box 210, Atlanta, TX 75551, 1988.

17. Sally Fallon, Pat Connolly, Mary G. Enig, Ph.D., *Nourishing Traditions,* Promotion Publishing, 3368 F governor Drive, Suite 144, San Diego, CA 92122.

Candidiasis: Scourge of Arthritics[29]
Introduction

According to the *Candida Research and Information Foundation Newsletter*[9], "The numbers continue to grow of people of all ages presenting with what has become an all too familiar set of symptoms who are told by their doctors to see a psychiatrist, to grow up, to have an affair, to go get a job, or simply laughed out of the office . . . among the many stories. . . there is indeed a problem —a serious problem . . . affecting the young and the elderly and all age groups in between."

The article, of course, is speaking of the wide-spread, modern disease known as Candidiasis and also known as monilia when found in the mouth.

The fact that arthritics' immunological systems are not working properly has led medical research, through pharmaceutical companies, to search for a means of "modulating" the immuological system. All arthritics do, indeed, have something wrong with their immunological system, but this is hardly a logical reason for further damaging it by means of cytotoxic drugs, gold, penicillamine or long-term corticosteroids. Indeed, this is also not a scientific rationale for assuming that the cause of Rheumatoid Disease is because of the obviously weakened immunological system.

Heavy use of antiobiotics will knock out the "good guys" microflora in our intestinal tracts, and that fact in turn permits organisms of opportunity, such as the ever-present yeast organism *Candida albicans* to take over. The disease that results, Candidiasis, is not yet recognized by orthodox medical practitioners, but its symptoms and effects are becoming ever more obvious to all. Whether or not the only cause for Chronic Fatigue Syndrome is *Candida albicans* is not known, but that it is a major cause of the symptomology can be readily assumed based on improvement that follows when Candidiasis is treated against. Even less known by established medical practitioners is that "vaginal candidiasis does not occur naturally without concomitant of *Candida albicans* within the large bowel and that a "cure" is not likely as long as the vagina remains the only treatment target[25]." It bears repeating several times: a vaginal yeast infection is an outward sign of a system-wide invasion.

According to Raymond Keith Brown, M.D., "Candidal infections, by depressing T lymphocytes can reverse T4 /T8 lymphocyte ratios, independently of the presence of the AIDS virus.

"Candida's presence, normally contained on skin, mucous membranes, or in the bowel, can be compromised by immunodeficient states usually induced by diabetes, pregnancy, or certain drugs. The latter include antibiotics, steroids, birth control pills, and chemotherapy. Thrush, common in infants before the full development of their immune systems, is frequent in immunocompromised individuals, regardless of their AIDS status.

"Chronic and often undetected, candidal infections are regularly associated with symptoms linked to every system of the body. Yeast cells (which are normally harmless and found within the intestinal tract) can be compromised by antibiotics, acid-base imbalances, nutritional deficiencies or parasites, so that they lose their protective cell-walls. Invading and distorting the intestinal wall with mycelia (root-like projections), they disturb the absorptive capacity of the gut. Considered part of 'the leaky gut syndrome,' they allow multiple antigens and toxins to enter the blood stream and spread throughout the body. Food allergies, although seldom diagnosed, are tied to this aspect of gastrointestinal dysfunction.

"The presence of candida can increase the toxicity of staphylococcal infections by multiples of 100,000, thereby suggesting a strong association with toxic shock syndrome. The latter, one of the medical mysteries of the 1970's. . . .[23]"

According to James P. Carter, M.D., Dr. P.H, "Iwata in Japan discovered nearly twenty years ago that Candida species produce toxins. . . . injecting Candida toxin into mice showed that it caused immunosuppression, among other abnormalities. . . In 1977, *JAMA* published the results of a study done at Michigan State University on college students who had recurrent vaginal Candidiasis. The authors pointed out that it was insufficient to treat only the vaginal infection. They also recommended changes in diet and lifestyle and suggested back then (1977), that the infection may have some effects on the immune system[8]."

All arthritics, by virtue of their weakened immune system, suffer also from Candidiasis, or "organisms of opportunity" similar to Candidiasis. Arthritics who are presumed to already have a weakened immune system, and who are obviously suffering from Candidiasis, certainly don't need another factor to further stress their immune system!

Candidiasis also creates additional food allergies, over time. Therefore, in addition to, say, symptoms caused by the disease of Rheumatoid Arthritis, victims also suffer from Candidiasis and food allergies, both of which not only add their own disease burdens to the arthritic, but both of which may also produce additional symptoms that can mimic those of Arthritis.

As the latter two conditions, Candidiasis and food allergies, often go unrecognized by traditional practitioners, all symptoms are blamed on the disease called Rheumatoid Arthritis.

All Arthritics should consider as part of their overall "get well" program treatment against Candidiasis.

Candidiasis, a yeast/fungus organism that seems to be everywhere,was first defined (*The Missing Diagnosis*) as a set of manifesting symptoms or syndrome by Orian Truss, M.D. of Birmingham, Al[1].

William B. Crook, M.D. of Jackson, Tennessee popularized Truss's findings in his book, *The Yeast Connection*[2]. Other physicians have also added to the popularization, such as Morton Walker, D.P.M. and John Parks Trowbridge, M.D.[3], *The Yeast Syndrome*, Dennis

W. Remington, M.D. and Barbara W. Higa, R.D., *Back to Health*[4].

Subsequent investigations by many physicians seems to have verified Truss's findings, and slowly but surely it is being accepted by the ultra-conservative medical establishment as a properly defined and diagnosed disease.

Candida albicans, which is found most everywhere, invades various parts of bodily tissues, resulting in localized infections. Common sites of infection are the mouth as in infant Thrush, gastrointestinal tract, vagina, urinary tract, prostate gland and skin and fingernails and toenails.

Under normal conditions our bodies are able to resist this invasion, as it does other germs. However, whenever various substances weaken the immunological system, the yeast/fungus organism begins to spread, and in the spreading creates virtual havoc throughout the body parts and systems.

The yeast/fungus invasion may cripple the immune system so that it can no longer repel invaders. It can create allergies to chemicals and foods. It is believed that it invades the intestinal wall where toxins from microorganisms and protein molecules from your food enter the blood stream, being there recognized by antibodies as a foreign antigen. Because proteins are derived from common DNA (gene molecule) structure, each time a new protein enters directly into the bloodstream, it, too, can become recognized as a foreign invader, and thus a "crossreactivity" occurs, causing one to have increasingly more food allergies.

Yeast, remember, feeds on sugars and carbohydrates that easily convert to sugars. In turn, yeasts produce a series of chemical products as waste among which are acetaldehyde and ethanol. Ethanol is alcohol, and there are cases of people on record who have never drunk a drop of alcohol yet are daily inebriated. Acetaldehyde is produced as the alcohol breaks down and is about six times more toxic to brain tissue than ethanol. These two chemicals are probably responsible for the following effects, according to Dr. Orian Truss[1]:

1. Cell membrane defects, damage to red and white blood cells and other problems.

2. Enzyme destruction. Enzymes are the key to breaking down foods in the body so that they can be utilized as nourishment.

3. Abnormal hormone response. Hormones regulate your bodily functions.

Some of the symptoms caused by *Candida albicans* are these:

1. Allergic reactions.

2. Gastrointestinal problems: bloating and gas, diarrhea, abdominal pain, gastritis, gastric ulcers, constipation, and many others.

3. Respiratory system: sore throat, sore mouth, contribution to sinus infections, bronchial infections and pneumonia.

4. Cardiovascular system. palpitations, rapid pulse rate, pounding heart.

5. Genitourinary system: vaginitis, frequent urination, lack of bladder control, itchy rashes, etc.

6. Musculoskeletal system: muscle weakness, leg pains, muscle stiffness, slow coordination, and so on.

7. Central Nervous system: Headaches, poor brain function, poor short-term memory, fuzzy thinking and so on.

8. Fatigue is extremely common as impaired metabolism doesn't enable the body to get enough fuel and impaired enzyme functioning inhibits energy production.

9. Weight gain is common.

As can be observed by reviewing the above characteristic symptoms (which are not complete) many similar symptoms may "present" with Rheumatoid Disease. It is often difficult to discriminate between one cause and another as diseases operate on the same tissues, the same organs, producing similar symptoms, in similar ways.

I recommend that you read the books listed in the references. Rheumatoid Disease spreads with a weakening of the immunological system. *Candida albicans* spreads with a weakening of the immunological system.

Rheumatoid Disease as well as Candidiasis seems to lead to food allergies and other kinds of allergies over time.

Both diseases produce similar symptoms in many bodily tissues.

Both diseases are systemic in nature.

A Candidiasis victim does not necessarily have Rheumatoid Disease, but a Rheumatoid Disease victim almost certainly suffers from Candidiasis.

Candidiasis spreads with the use of almost any kind of surgery where antibiotics were used, or if you've been given antibiotics orally for any purpose you probably suffer from some degree of Candidiasis. Why? Because the antibiotics kill off the "good-guys" bacteria required in your intestinal tract for good nutrition, the yeast/fungus spreads, taking the "good-guys" place, and sending rootlets into the intestinal mucosa, and helping to age your total system. These "good guys," such as *Lactobacillus acidophilus*, need to be replaced[5].

Candidiasis is usually controlled through a combination of diet control and medicines some of which are prescription and some nonprescription. Usually the physician who suspects Candidiasis also attempts to strengthen the immunological system by one means or another.

It is important to replace the yeast in the intestinal tract with *Lactobacili* as well[5]. If you are to use one of our recommended prescription medicines, metronidazole, the human body cannot metabolize it, according to a research pharmacologist[6], and requires *Lactobacillus acidophilus* for its metabolization. Metronidazole is one of the widely used forms of nitroimidazoles for treating and curing Rheumatoid Arthritis.

Here is another reason to take it. *Lactibacillus acidophilus* helps digest food and especially milk sugar. Some varieties also synthesize vitamin B and some reduce serum cholesterol levels.

While increasingly mounting evidence is being accumulated by traditional medical practitioners that Candidiasis is a real syndrome, much controversy still exists. Allergists, immunologists, and gynecologists see this syndrome as a fictional one, probably because the manifestations are seen too often, the need for treatment too frequent, the testing for its presence and effect too inadequate, and because almost everyone suddenly has become an expert in its presence or absence.

Paul A. Goldberg, M.P.H., D.C. says, "In 1977 I was a graduate assistant at the University of Texas Medical Center (School of Public Health) in Houston, TX. I had the opportunity to observe many cancer patients at the M.D. Anderson Tumor Institute there. Many (perhaps most) had candidiasis. The candidiasis was not the cause of their cancer -- rather it was part of the lowered resistance that had likely contributed to the cancer itself. Most sick people have yeast overgrowth . . . but yeast overgrowth is not what makes so many people sick — rather it is their lowered resistance. So, as our population continues to develop more and more degenerative ailments, what do we do? As a culture, ultimately, in addition to treating the effects of our lifestyles (e.g. the yeast), at some point the way of life in this country led by so many folks has got to be changed in some very fundamental ways.

"Why do so many people with candidiasis never get well? Perhaps, as suggested, it is because of changing yeast forms, not strict enough diet, not enough time given to treatment, etc. — but it is also because the real resistance of the patient never has the chance to really increase.

"Rest, sleep, sunshine, peace of mind, a conducive healing environment, none of these things are provided. So — armed with only a few drugs, supplements, and diet, a few recover partially, but many stay ill[27]."

Testing for Candidiasis

Most "testing" for the presence of Candidiasis takes place by means of a questionnaire which the patient fills out and the questionnaire is then evaluated by either a physician or a medical technician. If a score of a predetermined criteria is reached, one is at risk for having the syndrome, otherwise probably not.

Usually the questionaire is based on some variation of detail of the following characteristics, as listed by Morton Walker, D.P.M., John Parks Trowbridge, M.D.[3] :

1. Feeling lousy all over, even after having had many treatments;

2. Cause of rotten feeling can't be identified;

3. Patient has had repeated courses of antibiotics;

4. Subconscious preference for foods made with yeast — bread, beer, wine, alcohol, and certain cheeses;

5. Craving for sweets and other sugar-containing edibles;

6. Insistent desire for refined simple carbohydrates — candy, chocolate, cake, cookies, soda pop, junk foods;

7. Discovery that sweets and simple carbohydrates give a quick pick-up followed by a letdown;

8. Low blood sugar;

9. Usually high preference for alcoholic beverages;

10. Usage of birth control pills;

11. Usage of corticosteroids or other anti-inflammatory or immunosuppressive drugs;

12. Multiple pregnancies;

13. Abdominal pain, vaginal infections, PMS, menstrual irregularities, discomfort during sex, loss of libido and/or impotence;

14. Athlete's foot, jock itch, fungus infection of finger and/or toenails, fungus infection of skin;

15. Feel more tired on damp days or in moldy places such as basements, cellars or working in garden; and

16. Discomfort in proximity of smoke, chemicals and/ or perfumes.

Usually a high score on listing made from these characteristics is a very good indication of suffering from Candidiasis.

There are accredited laboratories that perform accurate, objective testing for the presence of the organism.

Such tests may be done in two stages, the first called the Micro-ELISA technique that detects circulating levels of Candida antigens, Candida antibodies IgG, A and M, and immune complexes. In the second stage of the test, the patient's lymphocytes (white cells) are challenged with Candida to evaluate inhibition of lymphocyte multiplication by budding (blastogenesis).

Treatment for Candidiasis

There are a number of recommendations for the treatment of Candidiasis, most of them relying on diet, a particular fatty acid, or a substance damaging to the yeast organism but not to human cells.

The prescription drug, Ketoconazole, is used by some physicians. Some use combinations of the above, coupled with mechanical or other means for cleaning out the intestinal tract.

The probable reason for so many approaches is because some physicians see improvements by one means, and stay with that means, while others see improvement by other treatments, and so favor that means. What most physicians do not recognize is that *Candida albicans* has six switching mechanisms[10, and seven viable forms, the last being a cell-wall deficient form[11, 12]. While it is well known among microbiologists, that micro-organisms will change shape and function according to their surrounding environment (i.e., more acid or alkaline, et. al.), it is not very well known among establishment physicians; or, if it is known, it is handily ignored so far as development of appropriate treatments.

A person who is symptomatically infected with *Candida albicans* most likely has the organism spread throughout many different tissues in the body. As different tissues may very well provide differing environments for the organism, it follows that there will be many different forms of the organism throughout the body. For example, a cell wall deficient form, not being recognized by the host's immune system, will float around in the blood stream until it changes to one of the other six forms. The blood stream, then, would provide a constant foci of infection for the organism. If only the intestinal tract is treated — as many physicians do — then there will be a constant return of the organism after what appears to be a "cure" has taken place.

The reason that *Candida albicans*, and other organisms of opportunity, have so many switching mechanisms is because they, like us, wish to survive, especially so as a species. They've spent many millions of years "learning" how to survive.

It is because of the seven viable forms taken up by *Candida albicans* that a particular treatment produces (1) extremely slow patient response, or (2) no response at all.

This conclusion derives from 13 years of responding to telephone calls at The Rheumatoid Disease Foundation, and to reading and listening to many fine clinicians on the subject of Candidiasis, and is a personal opinion only.

My conclusion, therefore, has been that if Candidiasis is to be effectively and quickly treated, all forms of treatment should be used either at the same time, or in as quick a succession as medically possible. Some of these will be described in detail in what follows.

Ketoconazole (Nizoral)

"Carol Jessup, from the University of California at San Francisco, treated 1,100 CFS patients with the anti-fungal drug ketoconazole, and 84% of these patients showed significant improvement. All of her patients met the Centers for Disease Control's definition of CFS [Chronic Fatigue Syndrome][8]."

According to one medical doctor[8], Candidiasis was adequately treated in those patients who tested positive by the above described test within three months by use of the prescription drug, Ketoconazole, without any diet being required. He felt that it was "ludicrous to assume that one can 'starve Candida out' by avoidance of sugar, yeast and moldy foods." (Ketoconazole is not one of our recommended 5-nitroimidazoles used for Rheumatoid Disease treatment, despite similarity in name.)

The same physician reported that those who tested negative by the above test (about two-thirds of those who presumed they were affected by the disease according to their own questionnaire) actually suffered from other allergies, hypothyroidism, other infections, heavy metal toxicities (especially mercury) and various types of functional nonspecific disorders.

His conservative conclusion was that there are probably some patients with intractable problems who should at least be tested for Candidiasis and if found positive, given a trial therapy such as Ketoconazole.

According to Raymond Keith Brown, M.D., additional "conventional treatment for candidal infection primarily involves antifungal agents such as clotrimazole (Mycelex), administered locally for thrush and esophageal involvements, nystatin (Mycostatin) for bowel therapy, and . . . , Fluconazole, and Itraconazole, for systemic infections. To avoid the side effects of these agents, many practitioners use natural substances, herbals, homeopathy, and acupuncture as possible alternatives[23]."

Some physicians will place their suspected Candidiasis candidates on rather extensive, stringent diets sometimes lasting for a year or more along with various medicines both prescription and non-prescription. Usually the diet approach coupled with certain fatty acids that damage the yeast organism, but are harmless to human tissue, is used often in conjunction with Nystatin, also a substance that is harmless to human tissue.

A most complete description of the Chronic Systemic Candiasis problem and its treatment comes from a paper written for his patients by Gus J. Prosch, Jr., M.D.[13].

Gus J. Prosch, Jr., M.D. Candidiasis Approach
Chronic Systemic Candidiasis
The Fungus Among Us[13]

Every human being from the day of birth lives in a sea of bacteria. Infectious germs known as microbes swim throughout our bodies at all times. These microbes can live in our throat, mouth, nose, gums, Gastrointestinal tract, blood, bladder, vagina, and numerous other body tissues.

These microorganisms which may be bacteria, viruses, fungi, or parasites, are as much a part of every human being as foods and chemicals. Figuratively speaking, they are constantly trying to "eat us alive." In some people they succeed and death follows. Even if we die of causes other than infection, they eventually eat our physical remains. Only healthy cells, organs and tissues within our bodies can effectively defend against infectious microbes.

Microorganisms, whether they are viruses, fungi, bacteria or parasites do not usually cause illness until an individual's host resistance declines. "Host resistance" is a technical term that doctors use to describe the complicated mechanisms by which our bodies fight off infections.

One of the most important defense mechanisms is the destruction of invading germs by our white blood cells, known as leukocytes. These special blood cells actually eat the germs and make them harmless. However, before these white blood cells can even be manufactured in the body, there must be an optimum supply of vitamins, minerals, amino acids and fatty acids. Many of these nutritional supplements, as well as adequate trace minerals, must be available in our bodies in order for these white blood cells to be manufactured properly. If even a single amino acid or fatty acid is deficient or absent from the body, leukocyte production is decreased and may even stop. When this happens, host resistance within the body is diminished and an individual becomes more susceptible to infections of all kinds.

There is another "host resistance" defense mechanism that we need to fight off these microbes, as well as any foreign substance that enters our body. These substances are called antibodies. When our bodies are receiving optimal nutritional support, specialized protein substances known as antibodies are produced. They are also produced by the white blood cells and these substances are constructed from chains of amino acids (proteins).

Antibodies attack the invading germs and render them susceptible to destruction by other white blood cells. Any germ that enters the body always stimulates antibody production that is specifically targeted against that particular type of microbe and no other. Once the body has made these specific antibodies, the lymph cells (another type of white blood cell) can then reproduce them any time they are needed, provided there are optimum levels of amino acids, vitamins, fatty acids, minerals and trace elements, along with enzymes from which they can be constructed. Therefore, if your antibodies against the tetanus or lock jaw germs (the reason for tetanus vaccinations), for example, have been sensitized, you will more than likely remain free of tetanus even if you are exposed to the tetanus germ. In such a case, your "host resistance," which has been maintained by proper nutritional support, will be functioning properly.

It is important to understand, therefore, that in the real world in which we live, infectious illness occurs not because germs arbitrarily decide to attack our bodies, but illness from germs occurs because our nutritionally deficient, debilitated bodies permit these microbes to set up residence. In short, an opportunist germ is an infectious agent that produces disease only when the circumstances in our body are favorable.

Nutritonal deficiencies can severely impair the integrity of a healthy immune system. There are, however, other factors that are also critically involved in resistance to infection. The eating of large amounts of sugar or sugar containing foods, for example, paralyzes the phagocytic capacity (the eating up of germs) by our white blood cells.

Therefore, when you do not get your proper rest and/ or exercise, resistance to infectious invasion decreases and it becomes easier for you or anyone to become infected with different germs.

Similarly, severe stress, such as the loss of a loved one, exposure to various chemical irritations, anxiety, chronic food-chemical allergies, and even chronic constipation or diarrhea, are other factors that can influence your resistance to infections. Yet at the top of all these possible causes of poor health, specific nutrient deficiencies must be corrected before you can "get well." Traditionally, the standard medical treatment for any bacterial infection consists of the administration of some form of antibiotic. Chronic Candidiasis is not like a streptococcus infection that, with the appropriate antibiotic care, one can expect eradication of the organisms from the body for several years.

Typically, with most physicians today, very little or no advice is given to the patient concerning nutritional support for weakened resistance. And, although traditional treatment generally involves drugs and chemicals that may relieve symptomatic disorders, the use of drugs does not cure the underlying nutritional-metabolic deficiencies which are usually the fundamental cause of the illness in the first place.

Antibiotics are very helpful and necessary in treating certain kinds of infectious illnesses. We must never forget, however, that if the nutritional root cause of infectious disease is not treated, illness after illness may continue to occur and often become worse as time goes on.

We must also never forget that typical antibiotic medical treatment aimed at the symptomatic relief of infectious flareups does in fact sometimes produce serious side effects in the form of fungal disorders as well as suppression of the immune system itself.

What is Chronic Systemic Candidiasis

Candida albicans, a form of yeast, is present in all of us not long after birth. It lives in our intestinal tract and is a yeast-like organism which in the infective phase produces a condition called "Thrush" or "Candidiasis."

Most medical practitioners feel that in the absence of the overt or obvious signs of Candidiasis, which is the acute infection stage of *Candida albicans*, there is no concern about this organism; and because of this, chronic candida overgrowth has not been well recognized. Normally symbiotic bacteria (good germs), proper gastro-intestinal pH (acid and alkalinity balance) and the body's immune system keeps *Candida albicans* in check.

Candida albicans is also called an opportunistic organism, because when a human becomes severely debilitated or nutritionally deficient, or if the immune system is compromised, or if the normal defenses (skin, decreased white blood cells, etc.) are bridged, then Candida can invade the deeper tissues as well as the blood stream. Before today's modern technological advances, most physicians did not believe that Candida could invade the body tissues. However, with the AIDS epidemic worsening, autopsies on patients dying from AIDS (their immune system is totally destroyed) are showing invasion of this Candida germ in the brain, lungs and other body tissues. Because of this finding, many physicians are taking a second look at the Candida problem and they realize that the germ can invade body tissues and cause systemic disease. Doctors by the hundreds all over America are now taking another look at this problem and many are trying to learn more about how to treat this condition.

Most physicians now recognize that *Candida albicans* can grow out of control in the nurturing environment of the mucosal (lining of the intestine) surfaces. Rapid and sustained *Candida albicans* overgrowth can lead to the pathogenic and often debilitating condition known as "Polysystemic Chronic Candidiasis." This is the fungus form of the disease. This new form of Candidiasis demands recognition and treatment. Many patients with this new form have had their symptoms for several years (chronic) and the symptoms usually involve multiple organ systems (Polysystemic). Because the syndrome produces so many symptoms involving multiple organ systems, it has been labeled Polysystemic Chronic Candidiasis.

Candia albicans is capable of changing its anatomy and physiology as it grows in the intestines. If its growth is mild and not overwhelming, it remains a symbiotic (living naturally in the body), sugar-fermenting organism that may manifest itself in such common conditions as oral thrush or vaginitis. However, if left unchallenged, *Candida albicans* converts into an invasive mycellial fungal form whose rhizoids (fingerlike projections) penetrate the gastro-intestinal mucosa causing many types of disease symptoms.

When the mucosa is penetrated by these rhizoids, the absorption of vitamins, minerals, amino acids and fatty acids can be seriously compromised and will further lead to many additional nutritional deficiencies. This breakdown and penetration of the mucosa results in the release of *Candida albicans'* metabolic toxins into the blood stream, along with intestinal substances, including undigested cellular proteins. The results of such far-reaching toxic and antigenic assaults can lead to tissue damage and systemic effects that constitute Polysystemic Chronic Candidiasis.

C. Orian Truss, M.D.[1] told how a yeast-free special diet and antifungus medication helped many of his sick patients to get well. His findings have helped me to help hundreds of patients to health and happiness. He said that the Candida organism can increase its numbers during periods of stress or lowered immune potential of the individual.

It is well known that the use of antibiotics for a long period of time can increase the Candida population in the intestinal tract, as well as the regular use of oral contraceptive medications and other drugs.

The yeast-like state is non-invasive but when it changes to the fungus form, it is invasive into the body. Penetration of the gastrointestinal mucosa can break down the boundary between the intestinal tract and the rest of the circulation and allows introduction into the blood stream of many substances which may be antigenic. This may explain why many individuals who have chronic

Candida overgrowth commonly show a wide variety of food and environmental allergies. The incompletely digested dietary proteins can then travel into the blood stream and exert a powerful allergic assault on the immune system which is seen as allergy, even producing a wide variety of effects such as cerebral allergy with depression, mood swings and irritability being a result.

Dr. Truss found that the classic test for *Candida albicans* overgrowth, a stool culture, does not always pin-point the chronic infection problem. His experience suggests that a clinical trial of an anti-Candida program is best administered when there are symptoms suggesting Candida overgrowth. Relying upon stool culture information alone to assess the problem many times leads to a missed diagnosis.

Dr. Prosch said, "In my practice, I also use a simple urine test known as the 'Indican Test' to help me in diagnosing this condition. It has been shown that when the yeast overgrowth plugs up the villi of the intestinal mucosa, a gas known as Indole is formed and this gas is absorbed into the blood stream and carried out through the kidneys. Measuring this Indole in the urine gives me a fairly good indication that a person may be suffering from an overgrowth of Candida. This is not a specific test, and is not reliable to determine a patient's response to therapy. "When the Candida yeast germ changes to a fungus form it definitely weakens our immune system. Our immune system is also affected adversely by heavy exposure to molds in the air and by exposure to chemicals, especially when this exposure is heavy or continuous. These chemicals may include gasoline, diesel fumes and other petro chemicals, formaldehyde, perfumes, cleaning fluids, insecticides, tobacco, and other indoor and outdoor pollutants.

"When your resistance is lessened, you may feel bad "all over" and develop respiratory, digestive and other symptoms, including fatigue, nervousness, depression, muscle aches and genitourinary symptoms, and you are apt to develop sensitivity to additional foods and to numerous chemicals in your environment. Such allergies cause the membranes of your nose, throat, ear, bladder and intestinal tract to swell and you tend to develop nose, throat, sinus, ear, bronchial, bladder and other infections. "Because you develop such infections, you're apt to be given a "broad spectrum" antibiotic by a physician who really does not understand the Candida problem. Such antibiotics promote the growth of Candida and your illness may continue until the cycle is interrupted by a comprehensive program designed to decrease the growth of *Candida albicans* and increase your resistance.

"Since the immune system is involved in fighting Candida and other infections, as well as allergies, I have noticed that in many patients, as the fungus overgrowth becomes worse, a patient's allergies become worse, and thus a vicious cycle begins; and the only way to break the cycle is to get the fungus overgrowth treated, which allows the immune system to better fight the allergies. Therefore, when a patient begins treatment for this Candida problem the allergies usually begin to get better even though it is a slow process.

"Not to diagnose and treat *Candida albicans* is a serious error because I've found that it causes more misery among women and men than all other diseases combined. In fact, I call the condition the great mimetic, because it can mimic almost any disease, from eye infections or allergy to colitis, cystitis, gastritis, brain tumor, multiple sclerosis, [arthritis] and even insanity."

Symptoms

Symptoms may result when the yeast *Candida albicans* succeeds in penetrating the tissues. Some of these symptoms result from allergic reactions to yeast products entering the blood stream from the sites of tissue invasion, while others may be due to toxic mechanisms (nonallergenic).

Finally, in the intestinal tract and vagina, the toxins originate, at least in part, from the sites of tissue invasions by this fungus. The yeast toxins affect your immune system, nervous system and endocrine (glandular) system. Moreover, these systems are all connected.

Therefore, fungus toxins play a role in causing allergies, vaginal, bladder, prostate and other infections, as well as fatigue, headache, depression and other nervous symptoms.

Yeast toxins also play an important role in causing loss of sexual interest, impotency, premenstrual tension, menstrual irregularities, infertility, pelvic pain and other disturbances of hormone function.

Every part of your body is connected to every other part so that when fungus toxins affect one part of the body, they are also causing change in other parts. Therefore, many varied symptoms may occur in men and women, depending on which system or which body organs and tissues are affected.

Dr. Prosch said further, "In women, I've found that the most common symptoms include fatigue, headache, depression, bloating in the abdomen, vaginitis, sex and menstrual problems, memory loss and a feeling of cobwebs in their thinking. I also see quite often as symptoms of the fungus infection, muscle and joint pains, numbness and tingling in various parts of the body, as well as nasal congestion, irritability, crying spells, and hives or itching.

"Occasionally I see patients who have chronic constipation and/or diarrhea, along with PreMenstrual Syndrome (PMS), infertility and Mitral Valve Prolapse. In fact, I've noticed that over 80 percent of the women who have been diagnosed as having Mitral Valve Prolapse suffer from this overgrowth of *Candida albicans*.

"I've also noticed that women develop the fungus connected health disorders more frequently than men. This is probably due to hormonal changes associated with the normal menstrual cycle, because the changes promote fungus growth as does birth-control pills and pregnancy. "In women, the anatomical characteristics of a woman's genitalia makes her more susceptible to vaginitis

and urinary tract infections.

"Women also visit physicians more often than men. Accordingly, they are more apt to receive antibiotics for respiratory, skin, urinary and other complaints.

"In men, the most common symptoms I see are fatigue, depression, headache, irritability, memory loss, along with impotency and impaired sexual drive, bloating and abdominal pain.

"I often see men who also have jock itch and athletes feet, along with prostatitis, nasal congestion, skin problems, hives and itching.

"Men can also have bouts of severe constipation and/or diarrhea and I have noticed that over ninety percent of patients who have been diagnosed with Irritable Bowel Syndrome or spastic colon, suffer to a degree from this fungus overgrowth of Candida. This condition is more prevalent in men who take repeated courses of antibiotics or who consume lots of sweets, breads and alcohol.

"I become suspicious of this condition in any patient who is bothered with recurrent digestive problems, food and inhalent allergies, and especially those who are bothered by fatigue, depression and nervousness. I do not, however, think that the disease is transmitted back and forth from husband to wife, but I have not been able to prove this.

"When children receive repeated antibiotics, the friendly germs are wiped out and the yeast multiply and change into the fungus form. The toxins are produced which may affect the immune system, nervous system, respiratory system and skin. So children may also develop yeast-connected or fungus-connected health problems including diarrhea (and other digestive disorders), skin rashes, constant colds, recurring ear disorders and unusual susceptibility to chemical fumes and odors.

"Among the most frequently seen fungus related disorders in children are those affecting the nervous system. Common symptoms include irritability, hyperactivity, short attention span and behavior and learning problems. Moreover, the nervous system problems in some autistic children are fungus connected."

Treatment

Again Dr. Prosch advises, "Successful treatment of Candida fungus overgrowth must follow a four-pronged attack to be effective. All four modalities of treatment must be strictly adhered to, otherwise treatment will not be effective.

"I cannot emphasize this point too strongly and repeat, **that you must follow the treatment plan exactly in order to get the best results of therapy. If you want to get well, you must follow these four steps of treatment and if you neglect any one of these four important steps, your treatment will be either prolonged, or unsuccessful when these instructions are not carried out.**

"These four steps include (a) killing the fungus overgrowth with proper diet (starving out the fungus) and medication (killing the fungus), (b) nutritional supplementation and correction of vital nutrients to build the immune system, (c) establishing a normal good bacterial flora in the intestine by supplementing *Lactobacillus acidophilus* (good intestinal germs), and (d) avoiding antibiotics, hormones, steroids and allergic foods. Of course there are other things a patient may do to speed up the healing process such as receiving proper rest, developing an exercise routine and sometimes adding garlic, aloe vera, Pau D'Arco tea and other helps."

A. Diet and Yeast Killing Medication.

According to Dr. Prosch: "The purpose of the strict diet is to limit the type of foods that feed the fungus. These foods will be discussed in a later section under Diet.

"There are numerous medications that can be used to help eradicate the fungus. Some doctors use primarily Nystatin powder and this is an excellent medication for treating the fungus overgrowth. I don't routinely start my patients on this medication because it is quite expensive and usually patients have to be treated for years instead of months.

"I use a number of medications to treat the fungus overgrowth and some of these are more effective than others: Capryllic Acid, tannic stearates and albuminates, fatty acids and even extracts from certain plants and vegetables, as well as some homeopathic remedies.

"In addition, I have been recently introduced to vaginal prescription medications, but these are extremely expensive and I prefer treating my patients in a natural way without the use of drugs and chemicals that could be dangerous to some patients.

"With any drug or medication, however, it must be emphasized that the worst thing a patient can do is to stop the treatment before therapy is completed, no matter what medication is given. A common problem that I have experienced many times is that patients try to 'play doctor' with their treatment and after a couple of months of therapy, they begin to feel so much better that they think they are well and stop the treatment. It is impossible to get this fungus overgrowth under control until at least three or four months of therapy, and when patients discontinue the treatment, the remaining fungus that have not been destroyed will simply grow back and very often will build up a resistance to the medication that had been taken to kill the fungus overgrowth.

"Patients who fall into this trap are always regretful so I insist on emphasizing to the patient that they should never stop the treatment on their own without consulting me first."

b. Vitamin, Mineral, Fatty Acid and Other Nutritional Supplements.

Prosch advises: "In order to build a patient's immune system, we must correct any vitamin, mineral and fatty acid deficiencies because all patients who have the fungus overgrowth are suffering from some or many nutritional deficiencies. I have developed a special vitamin-mineral supplement that I make available for patients that I treat for this condition, that is yeast free sugar free and is prepared in a special manner to get the best results.

"I also must be sure all fatty acid deficiencies are corrected and I make sure this is accomplished by furnishing patients with supplements of the correct, necessary type of fatty acids.

"I also instruct the patient in the proper eating habits to make sure that they do not develop further deficiencies of these vital elements in the future.

"I also have to be sure that certain amino acid deficiencies are corrected and this is done by supplementing certain amino acids in the vitamin/mineral supplement as well as making sure that the patient is following the proper diet.

"The above measures are absolutely necessary to ensure that the immune system is functioning properly, and to also ensure that the patient gets well as soon as possible."

c. Establishing a Normal Gut Flora[19].

Dr. Prosch continues: "To build up the good germs in our gastrointestines, I routinely prescribe a special form of *Lactobacillus acidophilus*. There are literally dozens of different types of acidophilus on the market today and the majority of them simply do not work. I've searched the entire United States for available types of acidophilus and I now routinely make available to the patient the type that I am confident is the very best available.

"The type I use is a powdered form (absolutely essential), and it must be refrigerated, and it contains ten billion good germs per one-fourth teaspoon which equals one gram.

"I've chosen this product because of its potency, good quality and effectiveness. Although the claims and labels on many types of acidophilus look the same, there are many strains that are not effective and have low potency and low bacteriologic count due to storage and handling. The type I use has proven that it works and is effective.

"Acidophilus in capsule form is not effective because we must build up the good germs in the mouth and throat. Capsules simply bypass these areas.

"The proper manner to take the acidophilus is to take one-fourth teaspoon four times daily, mixed in a small amount of water and swished a few seconds in the mouth and then swallowed.

"The main bottle should be refrigerated.

"A good way to take the acidophilus when away from home is to get a small empty pill bottle or vial and after taking the morning dose, place one-fourth teaspoon of the powdered acidophilus in the vial. This should be carried with you, and at lunch time the powder can be dropped into a small amount of water and swished in the mouth and swallowed.

d. Avoidance Recommendations.

Patients are advised to avoid antibiotics in any form as well as hormones, steroids and foods that they are allergic to.

Quite often, some patients will get a secondary infection from some type of germ such as a sore throat and call me to find out whether they should take an antibiotic or not. If the patient lives in close proximity to the Clinic, I recommend that instead of taking an antibiotic, they come to the Clinic where I can give them an intravenous infusion that will kill most any germ, and thereby the patient does not have to take an antibiotic.

Some patients are prescribed an antibiotic by their Dentist when they have dental work done, and I prefer that when this event happens, that these patients come to the Clinic for an intravenous infusion.

"Of course, sometimes patients live a great distance from our Clinic and are unable to come in for this injection. In such situations where they may have to take an antibiotic anyhow, I recommend that they take at least one-half teaspoon of acidophilus every time they take an antibiotic pill and also recommend that these patients take at least eight thousand to ten thousand milligrams of Vitamin C in divided doses each day. This will help to stimulate the immune system as well as to build up good germs that the antibiotic would be killing.

"As far as hormones, or steroids are concerned, I prefer that patients not take the substances, but sometimes patients must continue taking these medications, and I have found that we can usually get the patient's fungus overgrowth under control even though taking these medications, but it does take longer.

"Should the patient have any questions concerning the item, I ask them to discuss it with me during their visit."

Discussion

The most striking characteristic of the clinical picture of Polysystemic Chronic Candidiasis is its complexity. The erratic function in many organs is evidenced by appropriate symptoms. Particularly, those originating in the central nervous system, the GI, and GU tracts, endocrine glands, skin, mucous membranes, muscles and joints, and respiratory system.

To those hearing of Candidiasis for the first time, this very complexity of it's manifestation is perhaps the most single obstacle to acceptance of the concept that Polysystemic Chronic Candidiasis may be responsible for chronic illness. The objection voiced most often is that nothing could cause such multi-system illness. This reaction is understandable if human illness is viewed primarily in terms of individual organs and systems, and categorized as heart trouble, liver disease, kidney disease, stomach trouble, etc.

There are several other problems which occur at a frequency greater than expected in the general population to those suf ferin g from Polysystemic Chronic Candidiasis.

The first of these is mitral valve prolapse with dysautonomia. The medical history usually reveals that the symptoms on which these diagnoses were based had their beginning after typical symptoms of mold sensitivity had been present for several years. If we assume that these conditions are being diagnosed with reasonable accuracy, there has been a sharp increase in their incidence and it has paralleled the similar increase that has occurred in chronic fungus infections since the advent of broad spectrum antibiotics, birth control pills and steroid hormones.

Prosch further advises: "As for the overgrowth of the fungus form of the Candida, we do know that a chemical called acetaldehyde is formed and this can have an effect on collagen (connective tissue) metabolism. This, I'm sure, is in some way related to the mitral valve prolapse problems and it may also be related to an increase of a condition called Carpal Tunnel Syndrome, which I'm seeing more frequently.

"I'm also finding that many patients exhibit extreme intolerance to formaldehyde. Many companies in the home construction business are using formaldehyde in glues for plywood and paneling boards, etc. and this problem seems to be getting worse.

"Occasionally patients date the onset of their Candidiasis to heavy formaldehyde exposure. Along with this, allergic reactions to products of *Candida albicans* occur frequently due to the antigens of this fungus. Allergic rhinitis and asthma are not uncommon and chronic idiopathic urticaria (hives) is frequently due to the antigens of this fungus.

"Allergy to pollen, other inhalants and foods may appear in quick succession soon after the onset of chronic fungus infections, and on occasion may disappear abruptly with no therapy other than yeast suppression -- this suggests a relationship between *Candida albicans* and the unknown changes in the immune system that allow or cause allergic reactions to occur."

Once therapy is initiated, the symptoms o f approximately one in five patients will worsen. This is called a Herxheimer Reaction[14]. Some doctors call this a "die-off reaction" and others may even call it a "healing crisis." It occurs when a large number of Candida organisms are killed off during initial stages of treatment, resulting in a sudden release of toxic substances that results in an immune response and intensified symptoms. It normally lasts no longer than a week and is frequently confused as an allergic reaction toward the therapeutic agents.

The use of nutritional supplements and therapeutics, as opposed to drugs, tends to lessen the intensity, duration and frequency of these symptoms. However, when symptoms are severe, treatment should be backed off to tolerable levels and built up over time.

When the Herxheimer is too severe, I usually recommend that patients cut the dosage of their medication in half for a week and then go back to the original dosages.

If symptoms persist, alternative options for treatment may be given. Patients should continue treatment for this condition for at least three to four months before stopping treatment. If treatment is discontinued before the patient gets the condition under control, all their symptoms will usually return.

After the fungus overgrowth has subsided and the yeast are killed down to a normal level (and this takes at least three to four months) the medications and supplements are gradually decreased over a period of six to eight weeks and the patients are allowed to gradually add previously forbidden foods to their diet.

Foods You Should Avoid In Your Diet
When Treating Candida Fungus Overgrowth

The Candida fungus grows on sugar and starch and high carbohydrate foods and is fed by gluten containing grains. Gluten grains include wheat, oats, rye and barley.

The fungus also grows and is fed by other yeast molds, and yeasty foods. It is known that yeast, molds and fungi crossreact.

When taken in food or even breathed in high concentrations, they trigger symptoms and diminish the body's resistance to Candida overgrowth.

Bathrooms and air vents should be kept clean and dry. Yeast molds and fungi should be minimized in foods.

Therefore:

1. Do not eat any sweets or desserts of any type and this includes products made with honey or molasses as well as any form of sugar or products listed on labels that end in "ose," such as fructose, glucose, maltose, lactose, etc.

2. Do not eat wheat, oats, rye, barley, or corn. Starchy foods such as rice, potatoes, buckwheat, beans and corn, should also be excluded from the diet while treatment is being undertaken. Two rice cakes each day are allowed, however. A bowl of oatmeal is allowed each day, if desired.

3. Milk (even raw) encourages Candida fungus growth. Try to avoid milk, and milk products, except butter and plain unsweetened yogurt and especially avoid any yogurt that has fruit or sugar in it. Patients on this program are allowed one glass of either sweet milk or buttermilk each day.

4. Yeast is used in food preparation and flavoring in all commercial breads, rolls, coffee cakes, pastries, cakes and this, of course, includes hot dog and hamburger buns, cookies, crackers, biscuits and pastries of any kind. You must be very careful with any flour products or even meats fried in cracker crumbs as well as all cereals. All beer, wine and all alcoholic beverages contain yeast and therefore must be avoided. You should also avoid

commercial soups, potato and corn chips and dry-roasted nuts. Vinegar and vinegar containing foods such as pickled vegetables, sauerkraut, relishes, green olives and salad dressings all contain yeast and should not be used. Don't forget that soy sauce, cider and natural root beer also contain yeast. Also, all malted products contain yeast, as well as catsup, mayonnaise, pickles, condiments, and most salad dressings. The citrus fruit juices either frozen or canned, usually contain yeast and only home-squeezed fruit juices are yeast free. All dried fruits such as prunes, raisins and dates contain yeast, as well as all antibiotics.

5. Yeast is the basis for most vitamin and mineral preparations. Nearly all vitamin and mineral preparations purchased at a drug store or from a large pharmaceutical manufacturer is loaded with yeast and should not be taken. If the patient has any doubts about other supplements I ask them to please check with me or my Clinic before taking them. Some vitamins purchased in health food stores that claim to be yeast free are not really yeast free and one must be careful or they can really aggravate your fungus overgrowth.

6. Molds build up on foods while drying, smoking, curing and fermenting. you should therefore avoid pickled, smoked or dried meats, fish and poultry, including sausages, salami, hot dogs, pickled tongue, corn beef, pastrami, smoked sardine or other fish that have been dried or smoked. You should not eat any pork of any type as pork is usually loaded with molds and yeast. Dried fruits, such as prunes, raisins, dates, figs, citrus peels, candied cherries, currents, peaches, apples and apricots should be avoided. All cheeses (including cottage cheese), sour cream, and other milk products, such as mentioned above,

should be avoided. Chocolate, honey, maple syrup and nuts accumulate mold and should be avoided.

7. Melons (especially cantelope and watermelon) and the skins of fleshy vegetables or fruits accumulate mold during growth.

8. Avoid canned or frozen citrus, grape and tomato juice. Avoid all canned or frozen foods which contain citric acid.

9. Mushrooms, truffles and many herbal products such as black tea, are loaded with yeast and should be avoided if at all possible. Don't forget that teas including herb teas and spices are dried foods and accumulate molds, so you should avoid these.

10. Eating fruit will boost blood sugar levels and will encourage yeast growth. But one fruit is allowed each day under this program, with the exception of melons and grapes. Bananas are probably the third highest sugar containing fruit and should be limited in amounts.

Be sure you read through this list of forbidden foods numerous times in order that you can familiarize yourself with what you can and cannot have to eat. Once you're familiar with these foods, it will enable you to select acceptable foods while dining in a restaurant or while visiting friends or neighbors at meal time. You should definitely learn those foods that you must stay away from if you want to get the best results in your treatment.

I'm sure you may be thinking "what else is there left to eat." We'll describe those, but meanwhile it is absolutely necessary that you carefully look at all labels on the canned and packaged foods and consult the above list constantly, or you will continue to suffer needlessly the consequences of the fungus overgrowth in your body.

Prosch advises: "You can eat out in a restaurant but order very carefully. Skip the cocktails. Have virgin olive oil and lemon juice on your salads. In fact, I routinely prescribe one tablespoon of virgin olive oil each day for patients being treated for Candida fungus overgrowth, because it not only has some good fatty acids in it, but the olive oil kills Candida.

"When dining out, order fish, chicken, turkey or lean red meats (other than pork) or other animal proteins that are prepared without sauces which might contain sugar, mushrooms or wheat as a thickener, and other harmful ingredients. Broiled or plain items are obviously the safest choice. Steamed vegetables are perfect but you must skip bread, crackers and desserts of any kind."

Remember, you must totally and absolutely avoid:

1. All sweets and desserts and sugar foods in any shape, form or fashion.

2. All breads and flour products (including whole wheat) of any kind.

3. All cheeses while on this program.

4. Any kind of alcohol beverages which are strictly forbidden since they contain sugar and yeast.

Candida Diet Allowables: What you Can Eat on This Program

Vegetables

Artichoke   Asparagus   Bamboo Shoots   Beet Greens   Broccoli   Brussel Sprouts   Cabbage
Caraway   Carrots   Catnip   Cauliflower Chickory
Collards Dandelion   Dulse   Egg Plant
Endive   Fennel   Green   Beans(Fresh)   Green Peas(Fresh) Kelp   Mustard Greens   Okra   Peppers
Rhubarb   SquashString Beans

Swiss Chard   String Beans   Turnip Greens Water Cress

To wash vegetables, use one tablespoon of bleach or clorox in one gallon of cool water.

<u>Salad Vegetables</u>

Alfalfa Sprouts   Bamboo Shoots   B r occoli Cabbage   Caraway   Catnip Cauliflower Celery Chard Chives Cress Dandelion Dulse Endive Fennel Kale   Kelp Leeks Lettuce Mung Bean Sprouts Parsley   Peppers   Rhubarb Spinach Squash   Swiss Chard Water Cress

Fresh tomatoes and onions are also allowed, along with summer squash and zucchini -all types of squash.

<u>Meats and Proteins (All Lean Cuts)</u> Beef Chicken   Clams   Crab Eggs   Ham   Lobster Salmon   Shrimp   Tuna Turkey   Veal

Also all game birds and animals such as squirrel, rabbit,   quail, duck goose and venison are allowed.

<u>Nuts and Seeds</u>

In limited amounts (one ounce) -- Walnuts, Sunflower seeds and Pumpkin Seeds.

<u>Oils</u>

Use only cold pressed or expeller pressed or non-hydrogenated oils. Also, you should take one tablespoon of virgin olive oil each day on your salads or vegetables. You can add lemon juice to this if you so desire. The best salad dressing is virgin olive oil in lemon juice.

<u>Other Items</u>

You may have two rice cakes daily.

Eat real butter and totally avoid all margarine.

You may have plain unsweetened yogurt but no yogurt with fruit or sugar in it.

140

You may have one cup of oatmeal (the old fashioned kind) per day. One small to medium fruit per day is permitted, but no melons or grapes.

You may have any unsweetened, decaffeinated drink. Any coffee you drink should be decaffeinated and your tea should be weak. If you must drink diet drinks they should be caffeine free and sugar free and you may have no more than two each day, maximum. You may have either

two packages of Nutri-Sweet® or Equal® or Aspartame®

as sweetners, but no more each day, whether they are in packages or in your diet drinks. You may, however, have Sweet and Low® or saccharine in any amounts you desire

. [Stephan Cooter, Ph.D. says that "It might be of interest to know that Aspartame or Nutra-Sweet, when metabolized, is half transformed into aldehydes responsible for the diet drink 'hangover': H.J. Roberts, *Sweet'ner Dearest*, Sunshine Sentinel Press, ISBN 0-9633360-1-5. *Citizens for Health Newsletter*, for instance, reported that the FDA had over 5,500 complaints against Aspartame in 1992, uncomfortably and closely related to worsening of Multiple Sclerosis and arthritic symptoms, tied to aldehyde toxicity": Ed.[22] (Aspartame is a nerve toxin that stimulates the appetite, so folks you think this is

a good drink for dieting are totally deceived.)

You may use salt, pepper, garlic or onions if you desire. Prosch adds: "For those patients who tend to lose weight easily, and especially those who should not lose any weight, I recommend that these patients eat three or four large tablespoons of homemade mayonnaise each day. "You must not use store bought mayonnaise as it contains hydrogenated oils. The mayonnaise recipe listed below contains 120 calories per tablespoon which will help prevent any excess weight loss by eating this each day. "Of course, if you are overweight you should avoid

this mayonaise. The recipe for mayonnaise is as follows: Take two fresh eggs, preferably at room temperature (take out of the refrigerator for a couple of hours before using) and add two tablespoons of freshly squeezed lemon juice (no bottled lemon juice) and add one teaspoon of salt (preferably sea salt. Mix this in your blender and add slowly one and one-fourth cup of cold pressed or expeller pressed or non-hydrogenated safflower oil." (One could use virgin olive oil or even coconut oil if you like the flavor.)

This is an excellently tasting mayonnaise and when refrigerated will last two to three weeks.

Don't forget that the diet in this treatment is absolutely vital and failure to comply with this diet will result in failure of treatment of your fungus overgrowth condition.

Stephan Cooter, Ph.D. would also remind arthritics that an additional screening of the Candidiasis diet may be necessary to avoid the Nightshade family, tobacco, potatoes, tomatoes, green peppers, and eggplant[22].

Medicines Used

Dr. Prosch used a variety of substances to kill *Candida albicans* overgrowth, among which are: Micocydin®, Paramicrocidin®, ParQing®, Borage Oil, SAM EPA®, *Lactobacillus acidophilus*, and various forms of Caprylic Acids and Olive Oil.

Most organic fatty acids are fungicidal. S.M. Peck and H. Rosenfeld demonstrated that Undecylenic Acid is about six times more effective as an antifungal agent than caprylic acid[26].

Candida Purge

William (Bill) G. Neely, D.C.[15] of Johnson City, TN successfully used a Candida Purge that contains a mixture of items to be used in a certain way, which will kill overgrowth while also helping to scrape fungal Candida from the intestinal tract. The mixture contains Caprol (Caprylic + Oleic Acids), Psyllium, Bentonite and *Lactobacillus acidophilus*.

The Caprylic Acid is fungicidal for *Candida albicans*. It is harmless to friendly intestinal flora, and effective against the invasive mycelial form as well as the yeast form, because it is absorbed by the intestinal mucosal cells. Caprylic Acid is metabolized by the liver and does not get into the general circulation. It must exert its fungicidal effect in the intestinal tract or not at all. According to studies, just ten minutes after oral intake of straight caprylic acid, more than 90% can be traced in the portal vein on its way to the liver. Consequently, Caprol should be taken with Psyllium Powder which will form a gel in the intestinal tract and release the caprylic acid trapped within over a period of time.

Oleic Acid (major component of Virgin Olive Oil: 56-83%) hinders conversion of *Candida albicans* yeast to the more harmful mycelial fungal form.

Psyllium gradually scrapes away *Candida albicans'* breeding ground (fecal encrustations) from the colon wall, absorbs toxins within the colon and carries them out, reduces toxic overload ("die-off reaction") from poisons released by dying Candida during treatment start-up and forms the gel which binds Caprol into a timed-release formulation. This powdered product gives slippery adhesive bulk to help loosen and dig out old, congested, solidified fecal matter that often coats the colon walls, thereby providing a breeding ground for *Candida albicans*, and other undesirable microorganisms. Because psyllium is not absorbed itself, toxic wastes are carried out in the feces.

Lactobacillus acidophilus arrests intestinal *Candida albicans* overgrowth, and is also effective against many pathogenic bacteria, thereby strengthening the immune system by lessening its workload.

Bentonite directly adsorbs *Candida albicans* and flushes them out, adsorbs toxins within the colon and flushes them out, and reduces toxic overload ("die-off reaction") from poisons released by dying Candida during treatment start-up.

According to Frederic Damrau, M.D.[16] "Bentonite is a native, colloidal, hydrated aluminum silicate. . . . It has been established in vitro and *in vivo* that hydrated aluminum silicate adsorbs toxins, bacteria and viruses. This property helps explain its therapeutic usefulness in acute diarrhea of diverse etiology. By virtue of its physical action bentonite serves as an adsorbent aid in detoxification of the intestinal canal."

Because bentonite is not itself absorbed, whatever it adsorbs is removed in the feces. This includes miscellaneous intestinal poisons, toxins generated by Candida (especially during treatment start-up), and the Candida itself!

Patients with severe Candidiasis (up to 50% of the cases) may experience certain uncomfortable effects within the first week after initiation of the Candida Purge program at the intensive level of therapy, such symptoms as flu symptoms[14] (stuffiness, headache, general aches, diarrhea) skin rashes, and vaginal irritation/discharge may result from the release of toxins from a rapidly dying *Candida albicans* population. The exact symptom picture

will depend upon the individual case and is often dramatic
— anything from "lead feet" to mental aberrations. The
exact symptoms are neither important nor do they lend
themselves to explanation, and they'll all disappear in a
few days, as also happens when the Herxheimer effect is
incurred in the successful treatment of other diseases[14].

Garlic, Aloe Vera, Pau D'Arco Tea

In the foregoing, Gus J. Prosch, Jr., M.D. mentioned
that there are other substances that can be used also, such
as garlic, aloe vera, Pau d'Arco tea and other items.

Garlic[20] is certainly an important supplement that
will speed your recovery by killing off *Candida albicans*
by preventing formation of lipids in the membrane of
Candida, thus obstructing the intake of oxygen.

The use of an odor-modified garlic extract (Kyolic®)
seems to shift lipids into the bloodstream, causing initially
higher serum lipid levels, but the lipids are then broken
down and finally excreted from the body, according to
Benjamin H.S. Lau, M.D., Ph.D.[20].

The use of this odor-modified garlic is dose dependent,
and over six months of daily usage, the good lipids, HDL,
increase and the bad guys, LDL/VDL, decrease.

Garlic has long been known as a natural antibiotic,
without damage to the "good guys" microflora, but now
Dr. Lau and many other scientists and physicians have
shown that *Candida albicans* drastically reduces in the
blood stream throughout six months of continuous usage.
More than that, however, is evidence that shows increased
protection from radioactivity damage, environmental
pollution, cancer protection, damage from stress, and it is
generally an immune booster, a nutritional supplement,
anti-oxidant, detoxifier, anti-clotting agent and anti-
microbial.

The studies by Dr. Lau were performed chiefly with cold-aged garlic preparations from Wakunaga Pharmaceutical Co., Osaka, Japan, but can also be purchased in the United States[20].

Aloe Vera has a number of attributes, among which is its antifungal effect against many pathogenic dermatomycoses[24]. Pau D'Arco, too, of course has many attributes besides its antifungal qualities.

Molybdenum Approach to the
Handling of *Candida albicans* Aldehydes

Dr. Stephan Cooter[18] wrote of a novel and new way to utilize the damaging byproduct of *Candida albicans*, that is, ethanol, and its descendant, aldehyde.

Dr. Cooter said that ethanol is not bad in itself, but when we receive too much of it, it converts to aldehydes. "If you have adequate amounts of glutamine, selenium, niacin, folic acid, B[6], B[12], iron and molybdenum, aldehydes continue to be metabolized into acetic acid, which can be excreted, or converted further into acetyl coenzyme A. If these nutrients are in poor supply, aldehydes begin collecting in the body's tissues.

"So when Candida is fully nourished (or we are), Candida furnishes the body with a necessary part of the Krebs energy cycle necessary for the health and maintenance of all cells. When our digestion is unbalanced, we incompletely convert sugars into poisons and they remain poisons in our human systems. When our digestion is balanced, or we give it what it needs in terms of supplements, a potential poison is transformed into a source of energy: i.e., aldehyde poison becomes acetyl coenzyme A[20]." The metabolic pathway described by

Dr. Cooter is that ethanol converts to aldehyde to acetic acid to acetyl coenzyme A. Cooter wrote that, "Within days of taking 100 mcg of molbydenum three times a day, I could feel the poisons from Candida garbage transforming themselves into heat and energy. Where I had experienced pain in my neck and shoulders, I felt warmth. A stiff back that felt like a wall of steel was transformed into copious sweat. My muscles relaxed and were pain free. At the same time, the person I was who found it difficult to get out of bed, became someone who needed only 4 to 8 hours of sleep rather than 10 or 12. Where I had been confined within a prison of fatigue, the fatigue was translated into an open expanse of energy and possibility. An intellectual fog that had filled my head for years scattered itself the first day I took molybdenum. I had lived with an aldehyde hangover for so long, I had no idea what it was like to experience mental clarity[18]."

Dr. Cooter stated that 100 mcg tablets of molybdenum amino chelate were chewed or sucked three times a day for 30 days in volunteer studies performed by himself and Walter Schmitt, Jr., D.C, with gratifying success for about two-thirds of the people who did try the supplement[18]. Their studies included changes in chronic fatigue, chronic weakness, joint pain, muscle pain, headache frequencies, mental concentration, depression, memory, and insomnia.

As Drs. Schmitt and Cooter have addressed the one problem that few other doctors have been able to find a solution for, i.e., the aldehyde poisoning caused by *Candida albicans*, they are to be commended. A candida treatment was also formulated under Dr. Cooter's name, called "Exspore." Dr. Schmitt's clinical findings were published in 1991, *Digest of Chiropractic Economics*,

31:4:56-63, and it was his insalivation protocol Dr. Cooter followed for both himself and the 31 people in Dr. Cooter's study. Dr. Cooter says, "Of special interest to me, was that Dr. Schmitt's discussion of aldehyde oxidase, the primary enzyme that metabolizes aldehyde into acetic acid and then acetyl coenzyme A, requires molybdenum for the conversion."

Drs. Henzi, Ponzi, and Schwyzer in Switzerland and Germany have also found, for instance, that B[12] and folic acid, provided a different metabolic pathway for the metabolism of formaldehyde in multiple sclerosis patients
(*Let's Live*, January, 1993: 66-68.)[22]"

We believe that the findings of Stephan Cooter/Walter Schmitt are well worth investigating for yourself.

Recommendation

Like the use of most alternative medicines, you and your physician will need to make up your own minds, especially after reading many of the books recommended.

This I know: The treatments reported here are generally safe in whichever forms they are offered to you, especially under a caring and knowledgeable physician interested in your welfare and in you as a personality, not a warehoused statistic. The treatments are generally low cost compared to other possible approaches. So, why not try them, if you fit the profile for Candidiasis. The trials surely will not harm you.

Virtually all Rheumatoid Disease victims are immunologically depressed — and Candidiasis grows well in such a deficient garden!

Many of the Rheumatoid Disease Foundation physicians use diet and special medicines to treat against Candidiasis along with our treatment recommendations for Rheumatoid Disease. Those same physicians seem to show a higher success rate in halting the progress of RD.

References

1. C. Orian Truss, M.D., *The Missing Diagnosis*, PO Box 26508, Birmingham, AL 35226, 1983.

2. William B. Crook, M.D., *The Yeast Connection*, Professional Books, PO Box 3494, Jackson, TN 38301, Third Edition, 1986, ISBN 0-933478-11-9. Also see *Solving the Puzzle of Your Hard-To-Raise Child*, Op. Cit. 1987, ISBN 0-933478-12-7.

3. Morton Walker, D.P.M., John Parks Trowbridge, M.D., *The Yeast Syndrome* , Bantam Books,1540 Broadway, New York, NY 10036-4094, 1986.

4. Dennis W. Remington, M.D., Barbara W. Higa, R.D., *Back to Health*, Vitality House International, Inc., 3707 North Canyon Road, #8-C, Provo, UT 84604, ISBN 0-912547-03-0, 1986.

5. Anthony di Fabio, *Friendly Bacteria* -Lactobacillus acidophilus & Bifido bacterium, www.arthritistrust.org, 1989.

6. Personal conversation with a Vanderbilt University pharmacologist, who does not choose to be identified, 1983.

7. Anthony di Fabio, *Psychiatric Pollution!*, www.arthritistrust.org 1989.

8. James P. Carter, M.D., Dr.P.H., *Racketeering in Medicine*, Hampton Roads Publishing, Inc., 891 Norfolk Square, Norfolk, VA 23502. p. 80, ISBN 1-878901-32-X.

9. *Candida Research and Information Foundation Newsletter*, No. 9-10, March 1989, PO Box 2719, Castro Valley, CA 94546.

10. David R. Soll, Ph.D., The Rheumatoid Disease Foundation *Second Annual Medical Seminar*, Santa Monica, CA, 1986.

11. Personal visit with Phillip Hoekstra, Ph.D., 1985.

12. Lida H. Mattman, Ph.D., *Cell Wall Deficient Forms*, 2nd Edition, CRC Press, Inc., 2000 Corporate Blvd., N.W., Boca Raton, FL 33431, 1993, ISBN 0-8493-4405-0.

13. Gus J. Prosch, Jr., M.D., *Chronic Systemic Candidiasis*, Biomed Medical Center, Inc., 759 Valley Road, Birmingham, AL 35226, patient handout sheet.

14. Dr. Paul K. Pybus, *The Herxheimer Effect*, www.arthritistrust.org, 1992.

15. William (Bill) G. Neely, D.C., 512 E. Unaka Ave., Johnson City, TN 37601, personal communication, 1992.

16. Frederic Damrau, M.D.,"The Value of Bentonite for Diarrhea," *Medical Annals of the District of Columbia*, Vol. 30, No. 6, June 1961, p. 328.

17. Nu Biologics, 2470 Wisconsin Street, Downers Grove, IL 60515-4019.

18. Dr. Stephan Cooter, "Molybdenum: Recycling Fatigure Into Energy," *Townsend Letter for Doctors*, 911 Tyler St., Port Townsend, WA 98368-6541, April 1994, p. 332; an excerpt from *Beating Chronic Illness: Fatigue, Pain, Weakness, Insomnia, Foggy Thinking*, Pro Motion Publishing, 10387 Friars Rd., San Diego, CA 92120, 1-800-231-1776.

150

19. Anthony di Fabio, Friendly Bacteria -*Lactobacillus acidophilus & Bifido bacterium*, www.arthritistrust.org, 1989.

20. Benjamin Lau, M.D., Ph.D., *Garlic for Health*, Odyssey Publishing, Inc., 2135 West 45th Avenue, Vancouver, B.C., Canada V6M 2J2, 1991, ISBN 0-941524-32-9. Also see:Tariq H. Abdullah, M.D., O. Kandil, Ph.D., A. Elkadi, M.D., and J. Carter, M.D., "Garlic Revisited: Therapeutic For the Major Diseases of Our Times?," *Journal of the National Medical Association*, Vol. 80, No. 4, 1988; Christopher L. Marsh, Robert R. Torrey, James L. Woolley, Gary R. Barker, Benjamin H.S. Lau, "Superiority of Intravesical Immunotherapy With Corynebacterium Parvum and AlliumSativum in Control of Murine Bladder Cancer," *The Journal of Urology*, Vol. 137, February 1987, p. 359; Benjamin H.S. Lau, M.D., Ph.D., Takeshi Yamasaki, D.V.M., M.S., Daila S. Gridley, Ph.D., "Garlic Compounds Modulate Macrophage and T-lymphocyte Functions," *Mol. Biother.,* Vol. 3, June 1991; Benjamin H.S. Lau, James L. Woolley,Christopher L. Marsh, Gary R. Barker,Dick H. Koobs, Robert R. Torrey, *The Journal of Urology*, Vol. 136, September 1986; Padma P. Tadi, M.S., Robert W. Teel, Ph.D., Benjamin H.S. Lau, M.D., Ph.D., "Anticandidal and Anticarcinogenic Potentials of Garlic," *Integrated Therapies*, School of Medicine, Loma Linda University, Loma Linda, CA 92350, 1990; address correspondence to Benjmain H.S. Lau, M.D., Ph.D.; Benjamin Lau, M.D., Ph.D., Garlic Research Update, Odyssey Publishing Inc. Op. Cit, 1991, ISBN 0-941524-32-9.

21. Wakunaga of America Co., Ltd, 23501 Madero, Mission Viego, CA 92691; telephone 1-800-544-5800.

22. Personal letter from Stephan Cooter, Ph.D., dated May 15, 1994.

23. Raymond Keith Brown, M.D., *Aids,Cancer and the Medical Establishment*, Trizoid Press, New York, 1993, ISBN0-9639293-0-5.

24. Dan Bensky, Andrew Gamble, *Chinese Herbal Medicine, Materia Medica*, Revised Edition, Eastland Press, Inc., PO Box 12689, Seattle, WA 98111, 1993, ISBN 0-939616-15-7.

25. "Candida Albicans," *Capsulations^{TM}*, No. 15, Thorne Research, Inc., PO Box 3200, Sandpoint, ID 83864, October 1989.

26. S.M. Peck, H.Rosenfeld, "The Effects of Hydrogen Ion Concentration, Fatty Acids and Vitamin C on the Growth of Fungi," *J. Invest. Dermatol.* 1:237-265, 1938.

27. Paul A. Goldberg, M.P.H., D.C., Personal Letter, May 18, 1994. 28. Boyd O'Donnell, "Laterflora `Raid'," *Townsend Letter for Doctors*, 911 Tyler Street, Port Townsend, WA 98368-7541, June 1994, p. 611.

29. Permission to publish portions of this article granted to *Townsend Letter for Doctors*, 911 Tyler St., Port Townsend, WA 98368-6541, January 1995, p. 64; permission granted to publish via internet, javilk@netcom.com, January 25, 1995.

Resources

1. Candida Research and Information Foundation, http://www.yeastinfectionnomore.com/Yeast-Infection-Candida-Video.php?hop=hatracker .

2. The Price-Pottenger Nutrition Foundation at 5871 El Cajon Blvd., San Diego, CA 92115. (Send a self-addressed, stamped, legal size (large) envelope with five

152

dollars and a list of physicians treating yeast problems will be sent to you.)

Allergies and Biodetoxification for the Arthritic

Food allergies contribute to Rheumatoid Disease. Even though allergies may simply cause a mimicry of the symptoms of Rheumatoid Disease, allergies may also help to cause the symptoms.

Food allergies are now classified in alternative medicine under the heading of Clinical Ecology, where the environmental causes of allergic symptoms are unraveled.

Certain allergy symptoms have sources that are well known, and easily found, such as those causing "hay fever" which springs from pollen or ragweed, pigweed, grass pollen, tree pollen and so on. This is an "external" allergy, as opposed to an "internal" allergy that springs from reactions to substances inside the body. External allergies do not usually cause symptoms of Rheumatoid Arthritis, but they can aggravate the condition.

External allergies can be discovered by the detective work of mixing together suspected allergens -- pollen grains, house dust, protein particles, et. al. — and after preparing the solution properly, inserting the extract just beneath the skin, where the size and severity of welts determines whether or not an individual is allergic to a particular protein.

Other external allergen sources — actually chemical sensitivies -- can be almost anything: gases, fluids, various proteins. Some people develop an allergy/sensitivity to something as common as the cooking gas from the cook stove, and they cannot live near or by such sources without being sick.

People range from very, very sensitive to not sensitive at all, in a gradient scale. People vary considerably as to what they are allergic to.

The interesting -- and distressing -- part about allergies is that foods which were perfectly safe for much of our lives suddenly become intolerable -- for no obvious reasons.

Early on in the medical history of treating allergies, professional allergists had great success in testing for and finding common allergens, such as from the pollens of various plants. However, when similar tests were developed for foods, or the increasing number of environmental chemicals, there was, at best, inconsistent results. Even today people will falsely take the skin-patch test which has shown itself to be negative, as proof that they are not allergic to the food the patch was supposed to test against. Food patch tests are extremely unreliable when making the determination for a food allergic reaction.

Since Theron Randolph, M.D. and four others organized the Society for Clinical Ecology in 1965 there has been a quiet revolution on how we view and test for food and other chemical sensitivities. By 1980 this society attracted 250 members. Dr. Randolph inherited some of his knowledge, and a great deal was his own major contribution to modern medicine.

There are claims, of course, that solving the food allergy problem will also solve the Rheumatoid Arthritis - - or other Rheumatoid Disease — problem. Some of these claims may be correct, and some may be, and most likely are, based on a mixture of three problems: Candidiasis, food allergies, and Rheumatoid Disease. More than likely, as we've suggested in other articles,

Rheumatoid Disease and Candidiasis go hand in hand, and then an increasing number of food allergies begin to also take over our health condition.

According to Paul Reilly, N.D. of Tacoma, WA, "Diet affects bowel flora and Gastro-Intestinal tract permeability. Both of these factors can, in turn, affect the amount of endotoxins (bacterial toxins released from dying bacteria) absorbed. In addition to their . . . role in stimulating B cell mitogenesis, endotoxins are potent activators of the alternate complement pathway, which promotes inflammatory processes. The Kupfer cells of the liver are integral in elimination of circulating immune complexes as well as antigens absorbed intact from the gut. If the liver is not functioning optimally, due to endotoxin damage, these undegraded antigens may be released into the systemic circulation where they can activate further complement release and inflammation[1]."

Allergy reactions also contribute to free-radical pathology, and that extra burden on the body can contribute to arthritic symptoms as well. After all, free-radical pathology, and subsequent damage, is what the damage of arthritis is all about. Cleaning up or preventing the development of extra free radicals, even temporarily, should give some relief, as seems to happen when using EDTA Chelation Therapy, DMSO Intravenous Therapy, or other similar means.

A most important publication to read and understand if you suspect that you're a candidate for multiple allergens from foods and other sources is *An Alternative Approach to Allergies*, by Theron Randolph, M.D. and Ralph Moss, Ph.D.[2]

Allergies, surprisingly enough, are also addictions, or at least there is sufficient commonality between the phenomena of food and some other allergies and addictions so as to suspect an actual biological link. Warren Levin, M.D. has contributed the following:

Allergy/Addiction to Foods and Chemicals
by Warren Levin, M.D.[3]

A new concept to the medical profession, but one of great importance to the healing arts, is food allergy/addiction. You will notice that I do not speak of allergy or addiction nor of allergy and addiction, but rather of a single entity — allergy/addiction. These two different aspects are as inseparable as heads and tails on a coin. Depending on which aspect is facing you, one or the other side may be more obvious but the obverse is always there.

Most of us are acquainted with the obvious food allergy reaction. The patient who breaks out from strawberries or swells up from shellfish or who gets asthma from peanuts is well known and recognized by the doctor or layman. However this type of acute reaction represents a very small percentage of all food allergy/addiction reactions.

The acute reaction occurs from exposure to a food which is not eaten regularly. The reaction may affect one or several organs or systems, but tends to affect the same systems in a particular patient with each repeated exposure. In other words, any organ in the body is capable of responding as the shock organ. If the nose reacts you get hayfever. If the lungs react, asthma. If the skin is the shock organ you get eczema or hives. If the intestinal tract is the responding organ you get diarrhea or constipation or nausea and vomiting or gas or a combination.

Allergy Causes Mental Symptoms

One of the most important shock organs that can respond to the allergic insult is the brain. The brain can show localized areas of allergic reaction similar to hives on the skin. Since the changes in the circulation, the localized swelling, the increased pressure of this allergic reaction are all taking place in the unyielding confines of the skull, the symptoms and signs of brain allergy can be severe or mild and manifest themselves as any physical complaint. The most common ones are headaches, fatigue, uncontrollable sleepiness at inappropriate times, inability to concentrate, memory lapse, incoordination, actual hallucination, changes in perception from any of the five senses — taste, smell, touch, sight and hearing. There can even be loss of consciousness and convulsions. The most important thing to understand about cerebral allergic symptoms (and I should say that cerebral refers to the most complicated portion of the human brain) is that these allergic symptoms can frequently mimic exactly the symptoms that have classically been attributed to nervous breakdown, neurosis or pyschosis. In other words the diagnosis that it's all in your mind may really mean that it's all in your brain and caused by an allergic reaction in the brain.

The most obvious example of a food addict is the alcoholic. Suppose we look at the history of an alcoholic from the point of view of allergy/ addiction. The first drink is almost always the social phenomenon. The drug affect of alcohol is experienced as pleasant and unwinding, the relaxation effect. This may be repeated socially at irregular intervals for years, without any addiction devloping. Then perhaps after a tough day at the office the businessman may try a martini before supper to obtain the same relaxation (still from the drug affect of alcohol.) When this becomes a habit the stage is set for addiction. Food addiction develops slowly from frequent repeated exposures to a potentially addicting substance.

It is at this point that the addiction phenomenon becomes manifest by its major clinical sign -- the withdrawal phenomenon.If you are addicted to something you feel better when you take it and after a period of being without it you begin to feel worse. Depending on the severity of the addiction it may be very mild and difficult to recognize, and express itself just as craving for the substance to which you're addicted. Some people just *know* that they are going to feel better if they have a cup of coffee, and other people just know they can't get started unless they have their drink of orange juice, and other people don't even recognize it — they just think that it's perfectly logical to have bread with every meal and they don't consider a meal complete without a piece of bread. What they don't realize is that the craving is to satisfy an addiction.

Withdrawal Symptoms Lead to Addiction

So let's look at our alcoholic again. He's been taking a martini now regularly when he comes home from work to unwind, and very subtly and gradually he becomes addicted. Every day by supper time his addiction is beginning to have its affect, and he relieves it by taking his customary drink. However when addiction becomes progressive the length of time that the offending substance relieves symptoms becomes less and less, and soon our harried businessman notices that somewhere around three thirty or four o'clock he is really beginning to feel frazzled. However if he keeps a little bottle in the drawer and takes a nip about three or three-thirty he can avoid that down feeling and of course it's an easy thing to do and that's only two drinks a day, and another alcoholic is on the way.

The addiction increases, the withdrawal period becomes sooner and now we find that in order for him to function well he's got to have a drink when he goes out with the boys at lunchtime. If he is intelligent he may skip the mid-afternoon nip from the drawer because he does not need that anymore but if he is a slave to habit he will continue to have that drink as well as the one before supper.

It's important to notice at this time that the patient is functioning better *with* the alcohol than he does without it, even though alcohol is a total depressant to the nervous system, interferes with reflex time and in general produces less efficient functioning. In the person with an alcohol problem the non-alcoholic state is no longer normal. It is a state of withdrawal from an addicting substance and the depression and malfunction that accompanies withdrawal is worse than the state in which the stimulation of the addicting substance is in effect.

Eventually, we get to the point where the patient is drinking every hour or two during the day to avoid the withdrawal syndrome, and he is functioning much below par but he does function as long as he continues to take his alcohol. However, now we see where the patient when he goes to bed at night, is going to go through an eight hour period and when he wakes up in the morning he's going to be in severe withdrawal. This of course is the classical evidence of addiction to alcohol — the patient who wakes up in the morning hung-over, nervous, irritable, and all he has to do is take a tiny sip of his favorite alcohol and he relieves withdrawal symptoms temporarily.

It is obvious to most people except the alcoholic that the best course of action is to go "cold turkey," to suffer through the withdrawal syndrome, to detoxify and then to avoid the offending addicting allergic substance so that optimum body function can be obtained.

In general we know that this detoxification or desensitization or cold turkey phenomenon takes about five days for food substances. What has been further recognized is that once a patient has gone through this cold turkey phenomenon and eliminated the allergic addicting substance completely, his body then no longer craves it and actually at that point becomes acutely reactive in an allergic way to the next exposure. This is extremely important in the diagnosis of food allergy/addiction.

It is important to remember that any food can be addicting. The best foods -- wheat germ, liver, yeast, meat, fish, fruit, vegetables — are capable of inducing allergy/ addiction just as well as the junk foods and alcohol. However it seems the more quickly a given food is absorbed from the intestinal tract, the more likely it is to produce the allergy/addiction response.

Fastest Absorbed Foods Are Most Addictive

Next in line to alcohol for speedy absorption from the intestinal tract are the refined carbohydrates like white sugar, white flour, corn syrup. In nature's foods the absorption of carbohydrates is slowed down by the presence of indigestible fiber, protein and oil. The refining process eliminates these factors which retard absorption and the result is increased incidence of allergy/addiction. The combination of these refined foods with alcohol is disastrous to the susceptible patient.

Following the refined carbohydrates in speed of absorption are the natural carbohydrates, fruits, starchy vegetables and cereals, then the proteins-meat, fish, poultry and eggs and finally the slowest of all — fats and oils. It is for this reason that many severely food sensitive patients are able to tolerate foods that are fried in oils Chinese style using the classical Chinese wok technique.

For anyone with multiple food allergies this method of food preparation is highly recommended.

The problem of identifying food allergy/addiction then becomes primarily dependent upon the recognition of the possibility. It's the old story in medicine — if a doctor doesn't think of the diagnosis during his contemplation of the patient he will never make a diagnosis. Once the possibility has been considered however, demonstration or confirmation of the correct diagnosis and treatment is straightforward. For in this case the diagnostic procedure is therapeutic -- that is, eliminating the offending substance from the diet will both demonstrate the allergy and relieve the patient. Many patients are skeptical even when they feel better after having eliminated their offending substances. For the skeptics confirmation is again an easy and straightforward procedure — one just says, OK, try that food all by itself and see what happens. Despite the fact that this procedure sounds so easy it is only easy in those situations in which the patient is allergic to one or a very few substances.

Unfortunately, many patients have mutliple allergies of varying degrees to many if not most of the foods that they eat. In such a situation eliminating a single food may not produce the relief that is sought and the withdrawal symptoms are merely super-imposed on the general depression and low functioning level, so that the patient feels worse and does not get relief at the end of the five day elimination.

Fasting Unmasks Allergies

It is in recognition of this particularly complex problem that the technique of total fasting has been developed as a diagnostic and therapeutic technique by the pioneers in clinical ecology. It is interesting to note that after many years of divergent pathways to health a number of different disciplines are finding that they have much in common. The religious ascetic frequently fasted to cleanse his body of impurities while he meditated, and noted that he was healthier in mind and body when he was through. The nutritionally oriented "health nuts" and some of the old time doctors and naturopathic physicians have advocated fasting as theraputic and detoxifying. Although the techniques of the various fasts have been different, the general concept is the same when viewed from the allergy/ addiction point of view. By eliminating all the offending allergic substances the body does begin to function at a more optimum level.

Needless to say, before starting on this procedure one should have the check-up and approval of his or her physician to make sure that the rare contraindications to fasting such as adrenal cortical insufficiency or Addison's disease and other debilitating illnesses are not present.

OK, so you're checked out and ready to start the fast. Just what does it mean to go on a total fast. Well it means exactly that, you are not going to eat anything, you are not going to put anything into your mouth except pure water, distilled water from glass bottles. The only thing that you drink is pure water without any mineral content — no tea or coffee made from pure water -- there will be no smoking either, smoking is one of the commonest food allergy/

addictions -- and that basically constitutes the fasting procedure.

The total period of fasting should be not less than 4-1/ 2 days. Some people continue to fast longer if they are tolerating it well and feel that they have not completely eliminated their toxic load. [It may take 5 days to clean all foods from the intestinal tract: Ed.] In general one should go into a fast expecting to feel worse before feeling better. The healthier the patient the less withdrawal reaction will be noticed. The more allergies and the more unhealthy the patient, the more severe would we expect the reaction to be. Usually if the patient's problem is primarily food allergy, the patient is feeling much better by the afternoon of the fifth day.

At this point we start refeeding the patient with the idea of avoiding a demonstration of an allergic reaction or the development of an addiction. That means the following rules are to be followed:

1. Initially after the fast eat only one pure food at each feeding.

2. The first few foods eaten should be foods that are not suspected of allergy or addicting potential to the patient. That means in general foods that are not in the usual daily routine diet. In some cases one must resort to exotic foods such as venison, bear or buffalo meat, kohlrabi, endive and rutabaga as vegetables. Goat's milk products are frequently acceptable. Remember that this is only in the initial phase of eating after the fast and eventually ordinary foods should be utilized for all but the worst cases.

3. If possible the first time a food is eaten after the fast it should be a fresh organic food known to be free of pesticides, preservatives or any processing. It is amazing how many people think that they are allergic to apples

only to find that it is the chemical spray at fault. Or an allergy to oranges turns out to be due to the artifical color and not orange itself. If there is no reaction to the organic product, the next exposure could be from the ordinary source of supply whether fresh, frozen or canned. I must add to keep my conscience clear as a nutritionist, that from my point of view everything we eat should be fresh and free of processing except as processed in our own kitchen.

4. Everything that is taken by mouth must be cleared of suspicion by individual tests. That means the first time you drink the tap water it must be all by itself. It is amazing how many patients are sensitive to the chlorine and fluorine and other pollutants in our water supply. It also means that every vitamin, mineral or food supplement as well as any medication must be independently judged by taking it and it alone and observing the effects. One of the biggest problems in the so-called neurotic patient is allergy/addiction to tranquilizers. In some cases to the medication itself, in other cases fillers in the capsule and frequently to the artificial coloring. However, you must beware of discontinuing any medication for the fast without your physician's knowledge even though any prescription can be a factor just as any food or food supplement can. Ideally nothing should be taken during the fast except distilled water.

5. Keep a diary with two columns. In column A keep an accurate exact record of everything you eat and the time that it is eaten. In column B keep a record of how you feel. Any change for the better or worse should be recorded with the time of the occurence. In addition keep a record of your pulse rate for one minute period before you eat each feeding and every ten to fifteen minutes for an hour

after each feeding. A change up or down of 12 or more beats a minute is suggestive of food allergy.

6. Continue eating single foods at each feeding until you have found a number of foods that do not produce reaction. After a few days of unusual foods start testing the most likely foods, the ones you eat regularly. Remember not to test complex foods like bread. This would be getting wheat, yeast, egg, shortening all at once. Test each ingredient separately. Foods for testing can be raw or cooked without any condiments or seasonings except for sea salt which may be used. Boiling, steaming, broiling and baking are the preferred cooking methods using the same water as for the fast.

Preservatives

One of the major problems that has beset mankind from its earliest efforts at civilization has been that of spoilage of food. Over the century the various tribes and races developed their own techniques for preventing food from going bad. Salting of meat, drying of grains, smoking of various foods, pickling in various ways and preserving in specially controlled temperatures and light are all included in some of the ingenious ways early man took care of this problem. However modern technology has come into the picture and with the ability to synthesize chemicals of great complexity, and in many cases to design a chemical to perform a certain function, food technology has become a billion dollar business and a very competititve one. From the original purpose of preventing spoilage we now have emerged into a cutthroat chemical competition to make the most brilliant colors, the most powerful tastes, the most artificial consistencies by modifying or in some cases imitating foods with chemical conglomerations.

The average child today eats a fresh strawberry and says "Oh, it doesn't have any taste," because he is so used to the intense artificial strawberry taste that he gets in anything he associates with strawberries; and the color of real strawberry is very pale in comparison with the garish pink of strawberry ice cream which is such a load of chemicals that I think it is a travesty to refer to it as ice cream. We are making people in this way get further and further away from natural food and dependent more and more on artificial colors, flavoring and the large numbers of preservatives. The important thing to realize is that all of these chemicals are frequent producers of allergic reaction and many people with long standing histories of erratic behavior, nervous breakdowns, hyper-active children are merely showing the results of the chemical sensitivity of the brain. It is certainly true that people can become allergic to the purest of foods from the harvest of nature. However, when people have these sensitivities they are much easier to handle when one is merely trying to avoid a food than when one has to consider the chemical problem as well.

Other Biodetoxification Regimens

Many different regimens exist for cleansing the body, and each physician will have his/her own favorite. Our chapter on Candidiasis, covers several other good mechanisms.

The use of body cleansing techniques is not presented herein as an either/or regimen, but possibly adjunctive to many other treatments that we have recommended or that your physician recommends.

References

166

1. Paul Reilly, N.D., "Natural Therapies for Autoimmune Diseases," *Townsend Letter for Doctors*, 911 Tyler St., Port townsend, WA 98368-6541, Issue #42, 1986, p. 331.

2. Theron Randolph, M.D., Ralph Moss, Ph.D., *An Alternative Approach to Allergies,* Bantom Books, New York, ISBN: 0-553-29830-6.

3. Warren Levin, M.D., "Allergy/Addiction to Foods and Chemicals," *Let's Live Magazine*, 444 N. Larchmont Blvd., Los Angeles, CA 90004, June 1976. Used with permission of Warren Levin, M.D.; Warren Levin, M.D., Anthony di Fabio, *Allergies and Biodetoxification for the Arthritic*, www.arthritistrust.org, 1994.

4. Major portions of "Biodetoxification" from Anthony di Fabio, *The Art of Getting Well*, www.arthritistrust.org, Op.Cit., 1988, p. 96.

5. Empty reference.

6. *The John W. Campbell Letters*, Vol. I, by Chapdelaine and Hay, (hc ISBN: 0-931150-15-9; pb ISBN 0-931150-16-7) and *The John W. Campbell Letters With Isaac Asimov and A.E. van Vogt*, Vol. II, 7111 Sweetgum Road, Fairview, TN 37062; (hc ISBN 0-931150-19-1); Also go to Kindle and Nook..

7. L. Ron Hubbard, *Dianetics: The Modern Science of Mental Health*, Bridge Publications, Inc., 4751 Fountain Avenue, Los Angeles, CA 90029, published from 1950 thru present.

8. 215. James R. Privitera, M.D., "Open Letter to the Wholistic community From an Old warrior," Op. Cit., *Townsend Letter for Doctors*, August/September 1992, p. 723.

9. Anthony di Fabio, *Chelation Therapy*, Supplement to The Art of Getting Well, Kindle and Nook, Op. Cit. 1993.

10. Efrain Olszewer, M.D., Alan Rory, Fuad C. Sabbag, M.D., Zapata, M.D., *DMSO (Dimethylsulfoxide) Treatments n Arthritis*, ; Ronald Davis, M.D., *A Treatment for Scleroderma & Lupus Erythematosus*; Supplements to www.arthritistrust.org, 1985.

11. American College for Advancement in Medicine, 23121 Verdguo Dr., Suite 204, Laguna Hills, CA 92653.

12. David W. Schnare, Max Ben and Megan G. Shields, "Body Burden Reductions of PCBs, PBBs and Chlorinated Pesticides in Human Subjects," *Ambio*, Vol. 13, No. 5-6, 984, p. 378. Also see Shields, Megan, M.D., "Hubbard Method of Detoxification Requires Niacin for Increased Effectiveness," Op. Cit., *Townsend Letter for Doctors*, July 1989, p. 378; Tretjak, Ziga, Shields, Megan, Beckman, Shelley L., "PCB Reduction and Clinical Improvement by Detoxification: An Unexploited Approach," *Human and Experimental Toxicology*, 1990, p. 235-244; Norman Zucker, M.D., "Hubbard's Purification Rundown: A Workable Detox Program," Op. Cit., *Townsend Letter for Doctors*, January 1990, p. 54.

13."Human Detoxification -New Hope for Firefighters," California Firefighter, Federated Fire Fighters of California, No. 4, l984, p. 7.

14. Foundation for Advancements in Science and Education, Park Mile Plaza, 4801 Wilshire Blvd., Los Angeles, CA 90010.

15. Zane R. Gard, M.D., Erma J. Brown, B.S.N., P.H.N., Giovanna DeSanti-Medina, "Bio-Toxic Reduction

Program Participants (Condensed) Case Histories," Op.
Cit.,*Townsend Letter for Doctors*, June 1987, p. 167.

Summary

This book *Rheumatoid Diseases Cured at Last* was
the beginning of The Arthritis Trust of America, legally
known as The Roger Wyburn-Mason & Jack M. Blount
Foundation for the Eradication of Rheumatoid Disease, Inc.

Roger Wyburn-Mason, M.D., Ph.D. was a world
renown nerve specialist, having had two nerve diseases
named after him prior to his death. Once he searched for
and seemed to find a cure for the more than one hundred
rheumatoid diseases, including rheumatoid arthritis, his
fellow physicians began to shun him. After all, if a disease
is "incurable" than no proper physician should claim that
it isn't. Such is the mind of the modern medical profession.

Dr. Wyburn-Mason claimed a one hundred per cent cure
rate of rheumatoid diseases. He and fellow physicians who
had actually tried his method could not interest those who
professed to be interested in curing victims of this scourge.
This foundation was begun to spread the news of a cure in
the face of strong negative pharmaceutical interests as well
as autocratic dictates from the general medical profession.

The Arthritis Trust of America (our present AKA)
began with the assumption that Roger Wyburn-Mason was
correct, that his treatment resulted in a one hundred percent
cure rate.

Not so! After trial by numerous alternative/comple-
mentary practitioners it seemed that fifty percent was the
best that could be expected.

Fifty percent!

Where presently only "immune system" modulators and pain relievers are offered to all victims with a 0% cure rate?

The following article, "How to Get Well" describes what we've learned since 1982. Getting well from rheumatoid disease of any kind is generally an easy chore -- except that to be sure of wellness the following treatment protocols must be explored and adhered to.

As a bonus, the same general treatments when sincerely tried will also bring about great relief — "cures" -- for victims of other allegedly "intransigent" diseases. What follows is a summary of everything we've learned since 1982. Normally one would not expect to engage all of the following treatments but surely, if you're a true arthritic, you'll want to explore as many as possible. That way ends with welness!

Cordially, Anthony di Fabio

How Do I Cure
My Rheumatoid Arthritis?
1. How Do I Cure My Rheumatoid Disease?

15 You start the cure by learning what Rheumatoid Disease is, where it's located in the body, and what causes it. The very first thing to learn is that it is a disease of the whole body, not of your joints. This is true no matter how much your joints ache or how insistent is your friendly neighborhood rheumatologist.

2. Where is Rheumatoid Disease Located in my body?

Rheumatoid Disease is a "systemic" disease. This means that whatever ails you is actually a problem of your whole body — cells, organs, systems — the whole works.

If you suffer from Rheumatoid Arthritis, for example, this systemic disease is manifesting itself in your joints. If you suffer from a differently named Rheumatoid Disease, then the target area of your body is given a new name, one different from Rheumatoid Arthritis. In fact, there are about 100 differently named diseases that have essentially the same causes but are known under totally different names as shown at the "Articles" tab, "Arthritis Classifications" at our website http://www.arthritistrust.org.

One of our founders, Professor Roger WyburnMason, M.D., Ph.D., explained this astounding fact by describing the medical profession's past technique for naming tuberculosis before discovery of the tuberculin germ. There were about 100 unique names for apparently different diseases depending upon the part of the body affected. Once the tuberculin bacillus was discovered, all of those names collapsed into TB of the bone, TB of the lung, TB of the skin, and so on.

We think Rheumatoid Disease is a cluster of symptoms named differently — 100 unique names — that can now be understood from the viewpoint of a single, systemic disease. (See "Arthritis Classifications" tab at http://www.arthritistrust.org.)

3. But what about my immune system? My doctor says that Rheumatoid Arthritis (or Rheumatoid Disease) is caused by a defective immune system?

There may be some folks who have a defective immune system, but these are probably rare. We believe that your immune system is doing exactly what it was constructed to do. By analogy, consider the camel with too many straws on its back. If you remove those straws one or two at a time eventually the camel will be able to stand again. Our recommended treatment protocol does exactly that —

removes the stressors from your immune system until your body (and immune system) functions properly again.

Professor Roger Wyburn-Mason again constructed a useful analogy citing past medical history. Prior to the discovery of the syphilis spirochete, the disease of syphilis was often considered a "defective immune system" disease. It displayed all of the characteristics of an immune system gone awry. Once the spirochete was found it was clear to all that this was an infectious disease problem.

Current internal medicine books will often provide two hypotheses for the cause of Rheumatoid Disease: (a) Something is wrong with the immune system, the body is attacking itself; (b) There is one or mor e microorganisms inside the body producing a reaction on the rheumatoid disease victim's tissues, thus causing the manifestation of the disease.

Billions of dollars worth of research following up the "something is wrong with the immune system" has never produced a cure. Whereas tens of thousands — stemming from the 1960s — have gotten well following up on the second, that is that the body is responding to one or more microorganisms.

4. What microorganism causes this terrible disease? Is there only one that affects everyone the same?

When we started the Arthritis Trust of America (The Rheumatoid Disease Foundation) in 1982 we believed that there was but one nasty microorganism, an amoeba. This was according to the findings of Professor Roger Wyburn-Mason and a world-class amoebologist, Dr. Stamm. Dr. Wyburn-Mason was convinced because his treatment designed on the basis of their alleged amoebic findings worked in the large majority of cases. We conducted numerous studies coming at last to the realization that Dr. Wyburn-Mason's treatment protocol was indeed working, but that his belief in an amoebic origin was not necessarily the best answer. (See *The Causation of Rheumatoid Disease and Many Human Cancers*, "Book s and Pamphlets" Ta b, http:// www.arthritistrust.org.)

Meanwhile, independently, Thomas McPherson

Brown, M.D. had concluded that a mycoplasm was the culprit in the creation of Rheumatoid Disease. (See "Thomas McPherso n Brown, M.D. Treatment of Rheumatoid Disease," at "Articles Important" tab of http:/ /www.arthritistrust.org.)

There are treatments predicated on both of these hypothesis, except that we've added additional, necessary wellness-serving treatment protocols. These are the necessity of correcting nutritional intake, anti-Candidiasis, learn food allergies,clean out root canal infections, get rid of mercury toxification, herbicide and pesticide accumulations, do hormone balancing, and so on.

We now believe that Rheumatoid Disease is caused by many factors (multi-factored) and that there can be one o r more out o f tens o f thousands o f invasive microorganisms to which a geneticall y sensitive person's tissues will respon d — either to the microorganisms' protein products or to their waste products. This is known as a "genetic susceptibility" to the toxins or protein products of the microorganism.

5. Should I have tests for these microorganisms, these pathogens?

Unless a health professional has some reason to search for a particular pathogen we feel it is a waste of money and time looking for any specific invader by the taking of blood tests or other traditional tests designed to find pathogens. However, Computerized Electrodermal Screening or applied kinesiology are two lowcost, often accurate means for making such a determination, if you wish to make the effort.

Experience has shown, however, that broadspectrum anti-microorganism treatment, coupled with investigation of all the other known causes and assisting treatments, is usually successful, at least 80% of the time.

Here's an example of a patient where our recommended anti-microorganism drugs did not work, but, by following our principles, the patient recovered from Ankylosing Spondilitis, one of the 100 or so named Rheumatoid Diseases. Reason: he was exposed to a whole different type of invading microorganism than normally found in the United States, *Schistosomiasis bilharzia*, a parasite obtained by swimming in Zimbabwe waters at an altitude where the waters are known to harbor this organism. He was able to get well by using the proper pharmaceutical created for this specific microorganism together with proper application of our other treatment recommendations — that is, unloading the immune system. (See http://www.arthritistrust.org. "Newsletters" "Spring 2005.")

We know patients who achieved wellness using only our recommended anti-microorganism treatments.

We also know of patients who only needed our other recommendations — not the anti-microorganism protocol — and got well.

Some patients require many or all of our recommendations to achieve wellness.

But, concentrate on the principles we describe and not on a literal-minded authoritarian approach.

6. How will I know exactly what to do? Take the anti-microorganism treatmen t or the other treatments?

Your best bet — if you truly want to get well — is to work with one or more knowledgeable health professionals, and to remove every single suppressor, every straw on the camel's back! You must learn more than your friendly neighborhood rheumatologist. This will be easy to do, because this group of professionals know absolutely nothing about how to get you well (according to their own statements), and you'll know something!

One drawback is this: There's no one health professional or dentist in the United States who offers all the treatment recommendations you will need to explore. Several clinics come close, but the majority of those who originally signed up on our physician referral list were rather limited in what they chose to offer you. So, if you truly want to get well, you should consider several options right at the start.

a. First off, learn everything you can on this website. Especially read the book *Arthritis* by Prosch and di Fabio at http://www.arthritistrust.org, "Books and Pamphlets" tab. Read it end to end.

If you don't understand some of the words, use "Google" or a dictionary or some other search engine to define them. Don't let words stand between you and a good understanding of the principles for achieving wellness. You won't have to learn your friendly neighborhood rheumatologist 's complex medical language, thank goodness, but you'll need to clear up some basic concepts to avoid confusion.

b. After you've learned as much as you feel you can absorb, then start searching for a health professional who will work with you. This could be your family doctor. We'll help her/him to learn, if s/he is openminded and willing to learn.

Otherwise, you can search for a doctor in your geographical region who is dedicated to or inclined to practice alternative/complementary medicine.

Plan on traveling to another location where exists a health professional who will help — and then plan on traveling to another location to visit another health clinic.

To find a biological dentist write or call **The Price-Pottenger Nutrition Foundation**, PO Box 2614, La Mesa, CA 91943-2614; (619) 462-7600.

Or, for a dentist, **American Academy of B i o l o g i c a l   D e n t i s t s** ; h t t p / / www.biologicaldentistry.org

To find a physician for allergies/chemical sensitivities/addictions **American Academy of Environmental Medicine** call (215) 862-4544)

To find a physician for heart/circulatory problems (chelation therapy) and many other problems write (self-addressed, stamped envelope) **American College for Advancement of Medicine** 23121 Verdugo Dr, Laguna Hills, CA 92653